S0-AAN-910

YOGA, TAI CHI

MASSAGE, THERAPIES
& HEALING REMEDIES

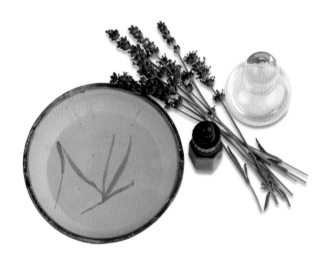

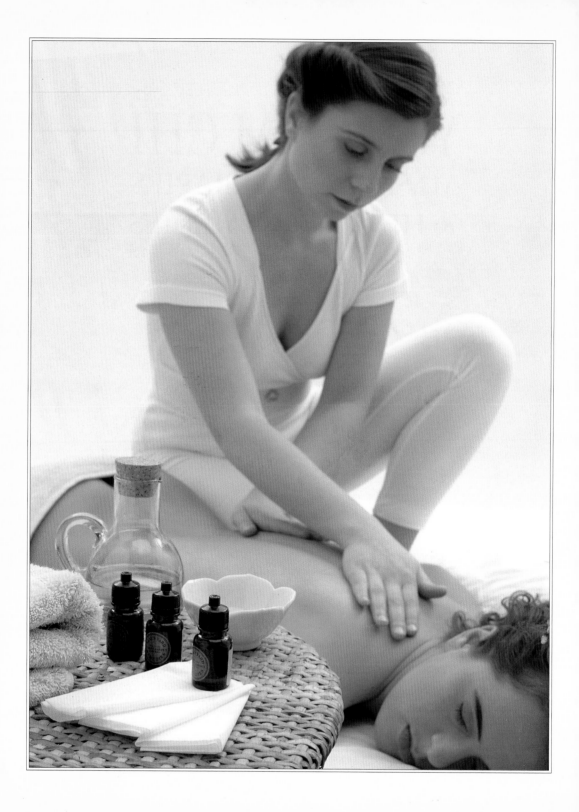

YOGA, TAI CHI
MASSAGE, THERAPIES
& NATURAL REMEDIES

natural ways to health, relaxation and vitality:
a complete practical guide

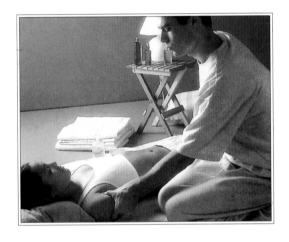

MARK EVANS B Phil., FNIMH

HERMES
HOUSE

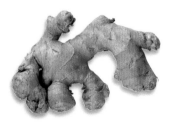

This edition is published by Hermes House

Hermes House is an imprint of Anness Publishing Ltd
Hermes House, 88–89 Blackfriars Road, London SE1 8HA
tel. 020 7401 2077; fax 020 7633 9499; info@anness.com

© Anness Publishing Ltd 2003

Published in the USA by Hermes House, Anness Publishing Inc.
27 West 20th Street, New York, NY 10011; fax 212 807 6813

All rights reserved. No part of this publication may be reproduced, stored in a retrieval system, or transmitted
in any way or by any means, electronic, mechanical, photocopying, recording or otherwise, without the prior written
permission of the copyright holder.

A CIP catalogue record for this book is available from the British Library.

Publisher: Joanna Lorenz
Editorial Managers: Helen Sudell, Joanne Rippin
Designer: Nigel Partridge
Photographers: Sue Atkinson, Simon Bottomley, Dave Jordan, Don Last and Lucy Mason,
Other chapters supplied by: John Hudson (Meditation), Michèle MacDonnell (Alexander Technique), Carole McGilvery
(Aromatherapy), Jimi Reed (Massage), Kate Shapland (Fitness and Exercise) and Paul Tucker (T'ai Chi)
Additional text supplied by: Andrew Ackroyd, Felicity Roma Bowers, Karine Butchart, Suzanne Franzen, Anne Gains,
Clare Harris and Paul Harvey
Exercise advisor: Dean Hodgkin

1 3 5 7 9 10 8 6 4 2

The majority of this volume was previously published as: *The Guide to Natural Living*

IMPORTANT NOTICE
The advice given in this book is appropriate in most cases. However, it cannot take into
account specific individuals' reactions. Neither the author nor the publishers
can accept any responsibility for claims arising from the inappropriate
use of any remedy or healing treatment. For further advice, and
before beginning any treatment suggested herein, read page 121 for
information pertaining to certain conditions and herb restrictions.

CONTENTS

NATURAL REMEDIES

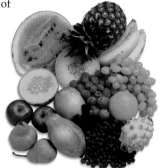

Health is, or should be, the most natural state of being. The origins of the word are linked with those of wholeness and healing, and it is that complete sense of harmony, of being whole, that brings true health. This is also the ultimate aim of the natural healing systems, those that adopt a holistic view rather than the reductionist perspective that is evident in much of conventional modern medicine.

In the last 10 years or so, there has been a great revival of interest in natural therapies, both as a recognition of their tremendous value and also as a move away from some of the side-effects and impersonal approaches of allopathic medicine. In this section of the book, we are looking at how natural therapies can be used at home, as self-help remedies, for a variety of common complaints; it should not be forgotten, however, that in professional practice more complex or chronic conditions can also be treated by alternative or complementary medicine, and if in doubt over any problem do seek qualified advice.

Many traditions of natural medicine extend back over several centuries, with an impressive accumulation of practical knowledge. For this section we have focused on four main therapies, which not only have such an established tradition but also have good standards of training, clinical research data and widespread acceptance. They are aromatherapy, herbalism, homeopathy and naturopathy.

Above: Fresh fruit is an excellent natural source of vitamins.

Opposite: Herbs can be grown successfully in ordinary garden flower beds, giving off wonderful scents as well as providing a useful source of herbal medicines.

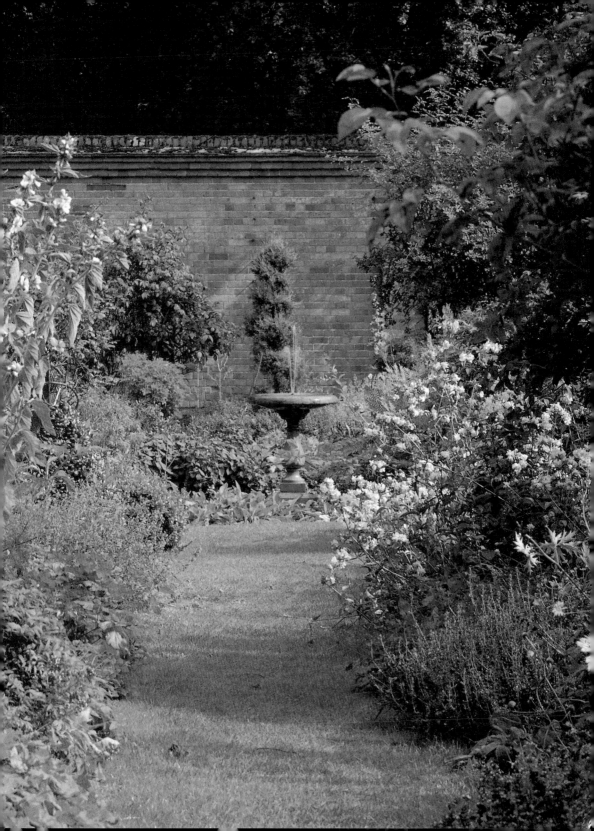

AROMATHERAPY

The use of pure essential oils from plants dates back many centuries, and the history of aromatherapy is in many ways part of the history of herbal medicine as a whole. The Arabic countries are credited with first discovering the process of distillation of oils, around a thousand years ago, and since then their use has spread both eastwards through the Indian sub-continent and westwards into Europe. Much modern research has taken place, for example, in France, ranging from perfumery applications to medicinal uses as powerful anti-infective agents.

Essential oils are highly concentrated substances – pure oil of Rose, for instance, may require 5,000 roses to make just 5 ml (1 tsp) of oil! For this reason they should be treated with respect and used sparingly – small is definitely better (and cheaper). In large doses many essential oils can become somewhat irritating to the skin, and a few are quite toxic if not used correctly. See general warning on page 121.

Since a large part of their effect on our moods and emotional states occurs through our sense of smell, it is important not to use any individual oil for too long, as they become tolerated and less useful. As a general rule, do not use an oil on a daily basis for more than 10 days. Similarly, do not inhale

Keep aromatherapy oils in well-stoppered bottles, out of the sun, when not in use.

Essential oils are very concentrated: add a drop at a time and only use the amounts suggested.

or mix too many oils together at one time; the olfactory centre in the brain becomes confused and an excess of essences can cause headaches or even nausea. Three or at the most four oils should be the maximum; two may be better.

A common way to use essential oils for self-treatment is in the bath. Place 6 drops on the surface of the bath water just before entering. The drops quickly form a thin film over the surface which adheres to the skin and is partially absorbed, helped by the warmth of the water. For oils such as Peppermint, which can make the skin tingle if used in large amounts, just add 3-4 drops, whereas with a mild and generally very safe oil such as Lavender, 10 drops can be used. If using a blend, the above suggestions represent the total number of drops to use in the bath. For compresses, use a maximum of 5 drops in a small bowl of hot or cold water as directed in this book (see page 15).

Another important method for using oils is diluted into a base vegetable oil and applied to the skin in massage. For home use a general dilution rate should be 1 per cent; since essential oils are usually sold in dropper bottles, this means a maximum of 20 drops per 100 ml (4 fl oz/½ cup) of base oil. Different cultures over the centuries have favoured various vegetable oils for massage, mostly dependent on local availability. Probably the most versatile oil is that of Sweet Almond; it is absorbed well into the skin and helps to nourish the skin, too. Other good base oils are Grapeseed, Sunflower and Safflower; the lightest oil of all is Coconut, but it may become solid at cool temperatures.

HERBALISM

Herbal medicine is the most widespread of all forms of medicine across the world, both historically and even today. At some time all cultures have used herbalism as the main system of treatment; its origins are essentially the origins of mankind itself. Probably the earliest herbal tradition comes from India. Medical knowledge from there spread into China on the one hand and into the Middle East on the other. The philosophy underlying Ancient Egyptian, and later Graeco-Roman, medicine has many similarities with both the old Ayur-Vedic system from northern India and traditional Chinese medicine.

Modern Western herbal medicine stems from the knowledge of the Greeks, with a strong input from the Native American tradition too. Increasingly, research being carried out today often confirms centuries-old empirical knowledge. Around 80 per cent of the world's population still relies on herbal medicine for their health needs, and even within conventional Western medicine up to 20 per cent of drugs are derived from plants in one way or another.

Herbs are almost certainly the most popular method of self-help in minor complaints, and introduce people to natural medicine. Throughout this book you will find references to how to take herbs internally; the easiest method is to make a tea, using a rough rule of 5 ml (1 tsp) per person plus the same for the teapot (many of the most popular herbs are available in tea bags, simply use one of these). If using fresh herbs, for example Lemon Balm (*Melissa officinalis*) you can use double the above amounts.

For stronger, more medicinal brews, you need to make either an infusion or a decoction (see page 12). For either an infusion or a decoction, the standard dose is 100-150 ml (4-5 fl oz/½-⅔ cup) – approximately a medium-sized teacupful – three times a day.

These infusions and decoctions can also be used to make a compress or poultice (see page 15). Once again, if using fresh herbs you can use more, perhaps 50 per cent more of each herb.

Many of the herbs found in gardens today have been used by herbalists for over two thousand years.

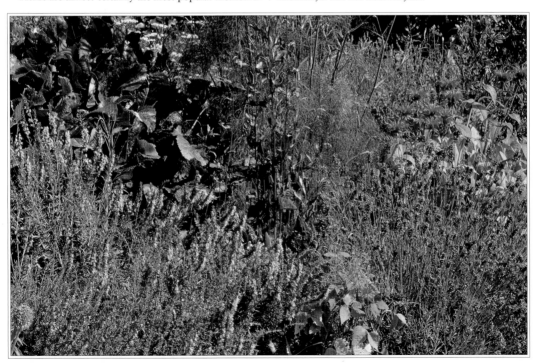

HOMEOPATHY

As a full system of medicine, homeopathy is much more recent in its development. It owes its modern origins to Samuel Hahnemann, a German physician, who formulated homeopathic theories in the late eighteenth century, although the principles were almost certainly known for hundreds of years before. Essentially, symptoms are seen not as negative effects of illness but as the attempts of the person to resist disease. Hahnemann tested a treatment for malaria on himself by taking many doses of quinine; after some time he induced malarial-like symptoms, and came to the conclusion that quinine worked precisely because it created these reactions in a healthy person; it mimicked and supported our own healing responses.

This led to the principle of "like curing like", and hundreds of homeopathic remedies have since been tested by giving them to healthy people and recording the responses. These "remedy pictures" are then applied to see which one fits the symptoms of an ill person. The other major point of difference between homeopathic and conventional medicine is that when a remedy has been identified as being appropriate to encourage the individual's self-healing mechanisms, it is then prescribed in minute amounts. Hahnemann had found that by diluting his remedies in a special way he was able to get a quicker effect, and he understood these dilutions to work on a more subtle level than simply obtaining a physical reaction.

One of the common scales for measuring the dilutions is the centesimal scale – that is, diluting the remedy in the ratio of 1:100. For a liquid this means one part of the remedy is mixed with 99 parts of a diluent, usually either alcohol or water. This is called a 1c dilution; this is then shaken in a special way, or succussed, and one part of this is added to 99 parts of the diluent to make a 2c dilution, and so on. As you can see, levels of extreme dilution are quickly reached, and so the remedy cannot be said to be acting physically in a conventional way, and indeed an important part of the "remedy picture" is the emotional reactions that are produced. The personality of the patient is a significant factor in choosing a remedy. Paradoxically, the more dilute the remedy, the more effectively it works.

A homeopathic practitioner may well use a very diluted remedy, to address an imbalance in our basic constitution, if there is a very clear picture that matches the individual.

For self-help treatment choose either the 6c or 30c potencies. For mild problems try taking the 6c dilution (normally remedies are available as tablets or pills, with directions for taking them with the container they come in) 3 times a day for up to 5 days. In more acute conditions, take a 30c dilution in the same way.

ACONITE
(Aconitum napellus)

In short-term, really acute conditions you can take up to 6 doses of either potency at 3-hourly intervals. Continuing to take the remedies for longer, however, may result in an aggravation of symptoms, as you "prove" the remedy in the same way that Hahnemann did. If in any doubt, and in any case if there is no response within this time, always see a professional homeopath.

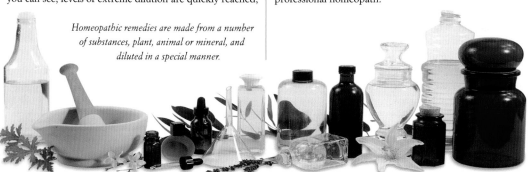

Homeopathic remedies are made from a number of substances, plant, animal or mineral, and diluted in a special manner.

NATUROPATHY

In many respects, naturopathy is really common sense applied to health. The basic principle is that we have tremendous innate healing abilities, and our systems will always attempt to overcome an illness and restore balance. In naturopathy, these attempts are encouraged by utilizing such natural factors as diet, exercise and relaxation, fresh air and the use of water (hydrotherapy). The general thrust of treatment is really to shift responsibility for health back to ourselves as far as possible, and equally to advocate prevention rather than cure.

Increasingly nowadays, ill-health is recognized as arising from environmental factors such as pollution, so an individual can only do so much to keep healthy, and wider measures may well need to be campaigned for. Nevertheless, a lot can be done through self-help action. While fresh, unprocessed foods are the main form of dietary treatment, there are times when this needs to be supplemented in order to raise vitality to a level where self-healing can take place, and so throughout the book there are some suggestions for supplements under different headings.

Exercise is a major form of self-help, obviously within limits of individual comfort. Both posture and correct breathing are an integral part of this, as effort without correct breathing can lead to strain. It is important to ensure that adequate rest or relaxation is taken too (easier to say than do in today's busy world!), and naturopaths would certainly give advice on these areas as part of the treatment.

The application of water by various methods, or hydrotherapy treatment, is another very useful part of naturopathy. The concept of using hot or cold water dates back at least to the Ancient Greeks, and is seen around the world in other old cultures, for example, that of Native Americans. Hydrotherapy treatment had a major revival in

The importance of regular exercise to keep our whole body fit, active and healthy is now well-recognized.

Europe in the nineteenth century, with the Bavarian monk Sebastian Kneipp the most influential figure. To this day, there are many Kneipp centres in Germany, Austria and Switzerland, which still prove very popular with patients. There are also around 120 different hydrotherapy treatments available in German health spas.

One of the simplest methods is to use a compress, or fomentation, made by wringing out a small towel in water and placing over the required area (see page 15). By alternating hot and cold compresses, – normally about 3-5 minutes if hot and up to 1 minute if cold – the local circulation can be strongly stimulated. For people who are considerably overweight it is often better just to use a cool compress, as this is less taxing on the heart. A shower can be used to similar effect by changing the temperature, or cool splashes of water after a warm bath may be used. A specific form of treatment in hydrotherapy clinics is the use of sitz baths, a kind of hip bath, which works on the pelvic and abdominal areas, by sitting firstly in a hot bath then transferring to a cold one for a short time, as indicated above.

As well as these approaches to health and healing, natural therapies range from those that work mainly via the body, such as massage, osteopathy, chiropractic and physiotherapy, through those that deal with energy balance, such as acupuncture, reflexology and shiatsu, to those that approach from the mental or emotional level, such as hypnotherapy, psychotherapy and group work. Each has its own strengths and weaknesses, and each attempts to help to restore balance from its own perspective. Some of them are not so easily applied for self-help, but it is useful to know that if you are unable to sort out your health problems on your own, then there is a wide choice of professional treatments that may help.

MAKING AN INFUSION

An infusion is made by pouring boiling water over an amount of the herb, to extract the properties. It is suitable for leaves and flowers, whose parts are easily extracted.

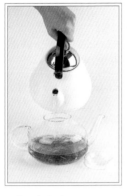

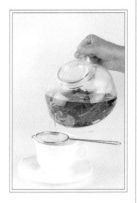

1 Place the herb in a teapot with a close-fitting lid. Pour in boiling water. Leave to infuse for up to 10 minutes.

2 Strain through a sieve or strainer into a cup. Store the remainder in a jug, preferably in the fridge.

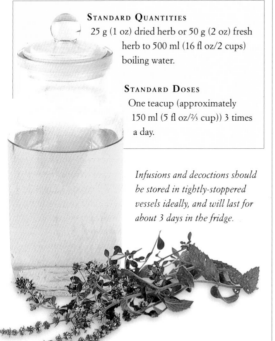

STANDARD QUANTITIES
25 g (1 oz) dried herb or 50 g (2 oz) fresh herb to 500 ml (16 fl oz/2 cups) boiling water.

STANDARD DOSES
One teacup (approximately 150 ml (5 fl oz/⅔ cup)) 3 times a day.

Infusions and decoctions should be stored in tightly-stoppered vessels ideally, and will last for about 3 days in the fridge.

MAKING A DECOCTION

A decoction involves simmering the herb in water to extract its properties, and is suitable for roots or woody parts that do not easily yield their ingredients in a simple infusion. If combining two plants, where one is a root, say Dandelion (*Taraxacum officinale*), and the other a flower, say Chamomile (*Chamomilla recutita*), use the strained decoction of the former for pouring on to the latter to make the infusion.

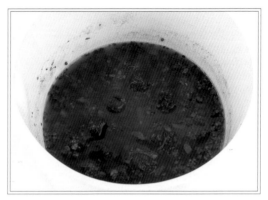

1 Place the herb in a saucepan and pour on cold water. Bring to the boil and simmer, until the liquid is reduced by a third.

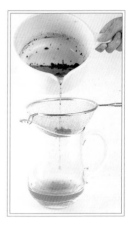

2 Strain through a sieve into a jug, and store in a fridge. It will keep for up to three days.

STANDARD QUANTITIES
25 g (1 oz) dried herb or 50 g (2 oz) fresh herb to 750 ml (1¼ pt/3⅔ cups) water, reduced to 500 ml (16 fl oz/2 cups) after simmering.

STANDARD DOSES
One teacup (150 ml (5 fl oz/⅔ cup)) 3 times a day.

MAKING A HOT OIL INFUSION

Herbs can be infused in oil, to make an extract for use in massage, or in making creams and ointments. Infused oils may keep for a few months, but will be stronger made in small batches for more immediate use. Hot infused oils may be made from herbs such as Comfrey (*Symphytum officinale*), while flowers such as Marigold (*Calendula officinalis*) or St John's Wort (*Hypericum perforatum*) are better as cold infused oils. Any light oil, such as Sunflower, Safflower or Sweet Almond oil, is a suitable medium to use.

MAKING A COLD OIL INFUSION

Some plants contain important medicinal oils which are highly volatile, i.e. they escape with heat, and a cold oil infusion retains their properties much more successfully.

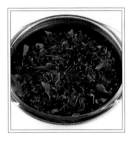

1 Place the herb and oil in a glass bowl, over a saucepan of simmering water, and heat gently for a couple of hours.

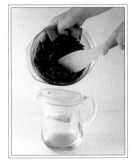

2 Pour through a jelly bag into a clean jug.

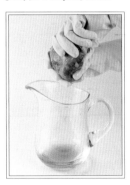

3 Squeeze out as much oil as possible through the bag (wear gloves as the oil is hot), to get a really strong extract.

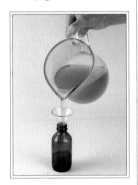

4 Pour into clean, dark bottles. Seal and store. Keep in a cool place and use within 3 months of making.

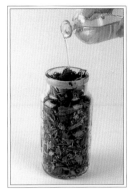

1 Pack a large jar with the herb and cover with oil. Seal and leave in a sunny spot for 2 weeks.

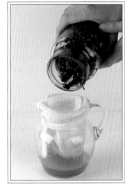

2 Pour slowly through a jelly bag into a clean jug, allowing time for the oil to filter through the fabric.

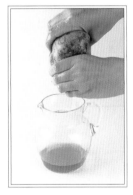

3 Squeeze out as much oil as possible through the bag. To make the infused oil even stronger, repeat steps 1, 2 and 3 with the same oil and new amounts of the herb.

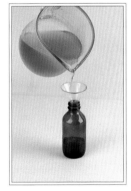

4 Pour into clean, dark bottles. Seal and store. Preferably, use small bottles as when opened the oil starts to deteriorate.

STANDARD QUANTITIES
250 g (9 oz) dried herb or 500 g (1¼ lb) fresh herb to 500 ml (16 fl oz/2 cups) pure vegetable oil.

STANDARD QUANTITIES
250 g (9 oz) dried herb or 500 g (1¼ lb) fresh herb to 500 ml (16 fl oz/2 cups) pure vegetable oil.

MAKING A TINCTURE

Many herbs contain active ingredients which are not easily extracted by water, or are destroyed by heat, and a tincture solves these problems as well as preserving the extract. A tincture is an extract of a herb in a mixture of alcohol and water, normally 25 per cent alcohol strength. This is one of the most concentrated extracts from a herb, and the alcohol preserves the medicine for 2 years or more. The alcohol used commercially is ethyl alcohol, but a spirit such as brandy or vodka can be used for home tinctures. Do not use industrial alcohol, isopropyl alcohol or methylated spirits, as they are all poisonous.

Because a tincture is such a concentrated extract, only use where recommended, and for short periods of time. Do not be tempted to increase the dosage.

CAUTION
If in any doubt about using a tincture, seek professional advice, or stick to the other methods described in this book. Do not give tinctures to children, unless advised, and remember to keep all medicines out of the reach of small children.

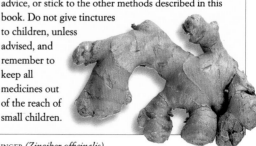

GINGER *(Zingiber officinalis)*

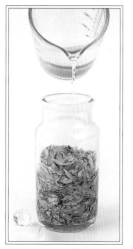

1 Put the herb into a large jar and pour on the alcohol/water mixture. Seal the jar and store in a cool place for two weeks. Shake the jar occasionally.

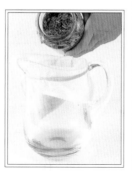

2 Pour mixture through a jelly bag into a clean jug.

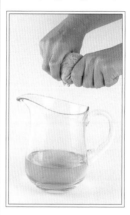

3 Squeeze out the tincture from the bag. Ideally, use a wine press and press the mixture into a clean jug.

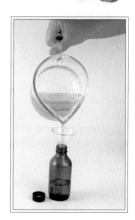

4 Pour the strained liquid into clean, dark bottles. Seal and store. Keep in a cool dry place and label.

STANDARD QUANTITIES
200 g (7 oz) dried herb or 40 g (1½ oz) fresh herb to 1 litre (1¾ pt/4 cups) 25 per cent alcohol/water mix (e.g. if using 40 per cent vodka or brandy, add 375 ml (13 fl oz/1½ cups) water to 600 ml (1 pt/2½ cups) spirit to make a 25 per cent strength).

STANDARD DOSES
Up to 5 ml (1 tsp), three times a day. These may be taken diluted in a little water. For concentrated herbs such as Ginger *(Zingiber officinalis)*, take up to 10 drops, 3 times a day. Preferably take these with water.

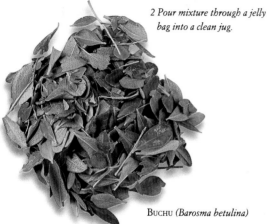

BUCHU *(Barosma betulina)*

WARM AND COLD COMPRESSES

A compress is a way of applying herbal extracts directly to the skin, to reduce the inflammation or promote healing. Usually, an infusion or decoction of the herb is prepared for use in the compress, or simply hot or cold water can be used.

POULTICE

A poultice acts in a similar way to a compress, but the herb itself is used, rather than just a liquid extract. Normally poultices are applied hot, and it may be useful to apply a little oil to the skin first, to stop the herb from sticking.

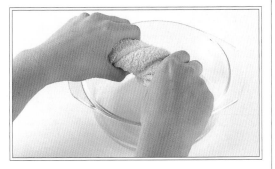

1 Soak a clean cloth or flannel in a hot infusion or hot water.

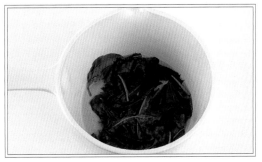

1 Chop up the fresh herb if it is too large, and place sufficient herbs to cover the affected area into a saucepan. Add a little water and simmer for a couple of minutes.

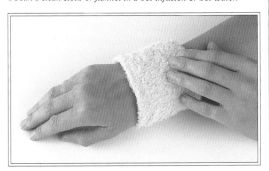

2 Place on the affected area and hold firmly in place – use a towel or bandage to tie in place if kept on for long. The same procedure applies for cold compresses.

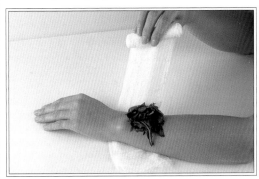

2 Squeeze out any excess moisture and place on the affected area. Cover with a bandage or cotton strips to hold in place.

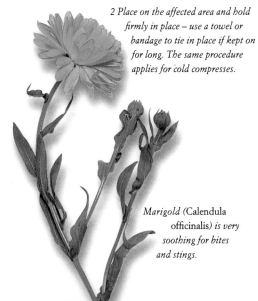

Marigold (Calendula officinalis) is very soothing for bites and stings.

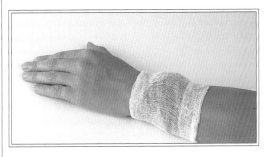

3 Keep in place for 3-4 hours, replacing every hour with a fresh, hot poultice if necessary.

MAKING AN OINTMENT

An ointment contains oils or fats, but not water, and is useful to form a protective layer over the skin. Petroleum jelly or paraffin wax may be used, but a wonderful natural method is to use vegetable oil, such as Sweet Almond or Sunflower, with beeswax. This is also very easy to make at home.

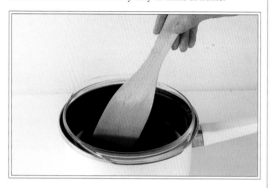

1 Place the beeswax and oil in a glass bowl over a saucepan of water. Bring the water to the boil and simmer until the wax has melted into the oil. Remove from the heat.

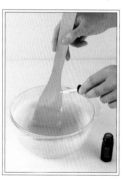
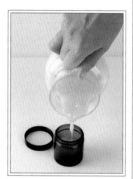

2 Stir continually as the oil/wax mixture cools and stiffens; essential oils may be added at this stage, as recommended, and stirred into the mixture.

3 Pour or spoon into small, clean ointment jars, seal and store. This may keep for a few months under good conditions, but should be made in small amounts as needed.

STANDARD QUANTITIES
25 g (1 oz) beeswax to 100 ml (4 fl oz/½ cup) vegetable oil. If adding essential oils, use 20-30 drops for this amount, but only 10 drops if skin is very sensitive.

MAKING A CREAM

Making an organic cream is very similar to making an ointment, again using beeswax.

1 Place beeswax and oil in a glass bowl in a saucepan of water (see left). Bring water to the boil and simmer until the wax has melted. Place water in another glass bowl, over a saucepan of simmering water. Remove both glass bowls from the heat.

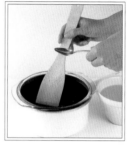
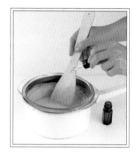

2 Add water to the melted wax/oil mixture, drop by drop, stirring all the time until the cream thickens and cools.

3 At this stage essential oils may be added, as recommended, and gently stirred into the cream.

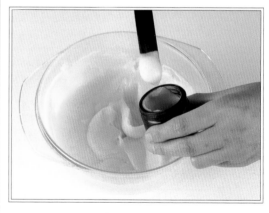

4 Pour or spoon into small, clean ointment jars, seal and store. Make small amounts as required. This cream may keep for a few months under good conditions.

STANDARD QUANTITIES
25 g (1 oz) beeswax, 25 ml (1½ tbsp) water and 100 ml (4 fl oz/½ cup) vegetable oil. If adding essential oils, use 20-30 drops at the most for this amount of cream.

MIXING ESSENTIAL OILS FOR MASSAGE

When essential oils are used for aromatherapy massage, different oils are combined to increase their therapeutic effect. Light vegetable oils such as Sweet Almond, Grapeseed or Sunflower are the best oils to begin with. For home use the general dilution rate should be 1 per cent (i.e. a maximum of 20 drops per 100 ml (4 fl oz/½ cup) of base oil). Once you have mixed your oils, store in a cool, dark place and use them immediately, as they are perishable.

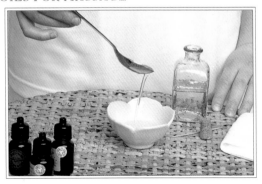

2 Gently pour the vegetable oil into your blending bowl.

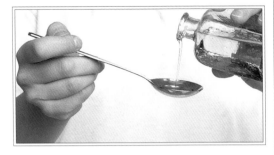

1 Before you begin, wash and dry your hands and make sure that all your utensils are clean and dry. Have your essential oils at the ready, but leave the lids on the bottles until they are required. Carefully measure out approximately 10 ml (2 tsp) of your chosen vegetable oil.

CAUTION
The essential oil recommendations in this book are extremely safe in the amounts given. If someone has very sensitive skin or lots of allergies then try massaging with just one drop of essential oil per 20 ml (4 tsp) of base oil at first to test for any signs of reaction (rare). If the person is pregnant or may be pregnant, stick to the oils and doses suggested in the chapter on reproduction. If in any doubt, seek medical advice.

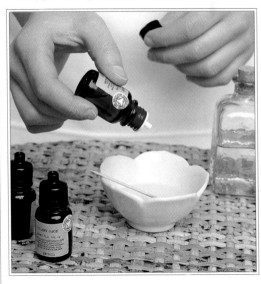

3 Add the essential oil, one drop at a time. Mix gently with a clean, dry cocktail stick or toothpick, to blend.

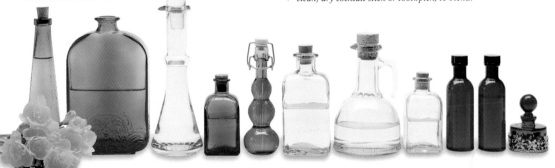

THE NERVOUS SYSTEM

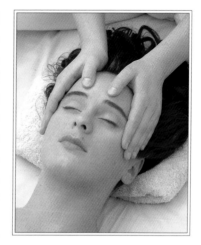

One of the main principles of natural medicine is the holistic approach, taking into account the physical, mental, emotional and indeed spiritual well-being of the person when assessing health; this is most obviously apparent when looking at nervous disorders. Physical symptoms, such as headaches or insomnia, and emotional ones, such as depression, mental strains and stresses, can all weave together to create disease, or simply *dis-ease* – a lack of harmony.

When trying to treat these problems, therefore, it is essential to look at all the reasons for the disorder. One of the first things to do is apply some common sense: is your headache due to an excess of alcohol last night, does your anxiety stem from tomorrow's interview, or your insomnia follow three cups of coffee in the evening? Finding the cause may not solve your immediate problem, but may help you to take preventive steps. In many cases of course, the causes are not so obvious and for persistent or recurring problems professional help should be sought.

Apart from the therapies described in this book, there are many sources of help for nerve-related conditions – since stress is a major factor in much ill-health nowadays, most forms of alternative medicine look at this aspect in their approaches. These might range from counselling and hypnotherapy through to acupuncture and cranial osteopathy. Equally importantly, these should all help to empower *you* to help yourself more effectively, which is the key aim of this book.

ABOVE: Taking time to relax and unwind is important for the overall well-being of our nervous system.

INSOMNIA

It is important to distinguish between habitual sleeplessness, repeated night after night, and a temporary problem due perhaps to some worry or anxiety. It is also important not to become obsessed with trying to get a certain amount of sleep; not everyone needs an 8-hour quota – quality is more vital than quantity. People generally need less sleep as they get older, or at least less continuously, so if granny has a day-time snooze and sleeps for less time at night, that is perfectly normal.

AROMATHERAPY

Essential oils are a very pleasant and effective means of unwinding and aiding restful sleep – try using them in the bath (see page 8) – or else putting 2-3 drops on to a paper tissue under the pillow at night. Choose from the following, either using a single oil or a blend; do not use the same oil for more than 2 weeks or you will find it becomes less effective.

CHAMOMILE: calming and relaxing in its effects, it is good where indigestion contributes to broken sleep.

CLARY SAGE: this has a sedating and almost euphoric action, *but* do not use if you have had alcohol as you can quickly get drunk, and have nightmares or a hangover feeling later on.

LAVENDER: not only very soothing, but also analgesic, so if any aches or pains contribute to insomnia, this oil is probably the best remedy.

MARJORAM: relaxing and warming, in large amounts it is quite sedating but can leave you feeling a bit thick-headed the next morning, so do not overdo it.

HERBALISM

An infusion (see page 12) of one or more of these relaxing herbs can help a return to a natural sleep pattern if stress has disturbed it. Other ways of using herbs include herb-filled pillows; traditionally hops were used as they are sedating (but not very pleasant-smelling!). Fill a small muslin bag loosely with the appropriate herb and place under your normal pillow.

Another old favourite remedy was cowslip wine; this not only tastes better than the infusion but is certainly very relaxing.

CHAMOMILE: *(Chamomilla recutita)*: calms the stomach and the brain, settling the digestion and helping sleep.

HYSSOP *(Hyssopus officinalis)*: a gentle relaxant; also helps to ease nasal congestion and colds, which can cause insomnia.

LEMON BALM *(Melissa officinalis)*: this helps to restore balance to the nervous system, and can be used safely on children. The fresh herb tastes much nicer, and can be drunk as a tea anytime.

LIME BLOSSOM *(Tilia europaea)*: mildly analgesic as well as calming; can soothe headache or other pains.

PASSIONFLOWER *(Passiflora incarnata)*: a strong relaxant or sedative, but without any ill-effects. Many commercial herbal tablets for insomnia contain this herb.

HOMEOPATHY

In the short term, look at these remedies:

ACONITE: for restlessness associated with sudden upset or fear, and resulting in tossing and turning in bed.

COFFEA: if the mind is completely awake and the brain will not turn off – just as if you had drunk strong coffee.

Probably the most versatile and useful essential oil is Lavender, distilled from the flowers.

NUX VOMICA: for insomnia due to overwork or excess food or alcohol, waking around 3 or 4 a.m. for several hours, with disturbed dreams.

SULPHUR: for over-excitement, with the mind full of ideas, and easily awakened by the slightest noise.

NATUROPATHY

In order to get the proper rhythm of energy through the day, it is useful to get plenty of exercise and get fresh air in the daytime. It may help to get up fairly early in the morning as well, to restore this balance. Do not sleep in a stuffy room, or drink coffee, tea or cola at night.

At bedtime, a calcium/magnesium supplement such as dolomite tablets can help to relax, especially if taken with a warm herb tea, or perhaps a hot milky drink if you do not suffer from a lot of catarrh.

MIGRAINE

Anyone who has experienced a migraine will know that it is more than a severe headache. Migraines generally involve acute pains, often over one eye, and perhaps disturbed vision or flashing lights. There may also be nausea or vomiting, and sensitivity to bright light.

AROMATHERAPY

Since the sense of smell is altered and often heightened during a migraine, aromatherapy is definitely best used between attacks; use at the earliest stage of a migraine only if the smell is well tolerated.

A central feature of the natural approach to migraines is to distinguish between a "hot" migraine, where the blood vessels are dilated, and a "cold" migraine, where there is excessive constriction of the blood vessels. In the first type, a cold or perhaps just cool compress (see page 15) across the forehead will give relief and oils of Peppermint or Lavender can be used. For "cold" types of migraine, a hot compress on the forehead or back of the neck may help, using Marjoram.

HERBALISM

Catching the migraine early gives the best chance of success (otherwise try to use these infusions regularly, as a preventive). Choose from the following:
CHAMOMILE (*Chamomilla recutita*): for dull, throbbing headache with a feeling of queasiness – add a little Ginger (*Zingiber officinalis*) to relieve more severe nausea.
FEVERFEW (*Chrysanthemum parthenium*): an excellent remedy taken daily to prevent the "cold" type of migraine, where there is a sense of a tight band around the head. This is widely available in tablet form as well.
ROSEMARY (*Rosmarinus officinalis*): good where stress is a trigger for migraines, and where local warmth gives relief.

CAUSES OF MIGRAINE

A migraine can be triggered by all sorts of factors: hormone changes, stress, stuffy atmospheres, noises, smells and certain foods are well-known triggers. Repeated attacks call for professional help; self-help treatments should be largely used as preventive measures.

HOMEOPATHY

During an attack try one of these:
KALI BICH: for an intense headache, preceded by a loss of vision and nausea, made worse in hot weather.
NATRUM MURIATICUM: for a severe, pounding headache with zigzags in front of the eyes, nausea and a pale face. The migraine may also be triggered by menstruation.
SILICA: for pains spreading from the back of the neck over to the eyes, usually right-sided, and often vomiting.

NATUROPATHY

Diet needs to be looked at carefully; try to avoid tea, coffee, alcohol especially red wine, red meat, cheese, chocolate, tomatoes and eggs. Eat plenty of fresh, raw salads and drink lots of fluid, as dehydration can be a factor. Try taking a Vitamin B supplement daily and see if this helps to reduce attacks. In between attacks, exercises to relieve tension in the neck and shoulders can be useful, and also massage of these areas (see left).

NECK MASSAGE FOR MIGRAINE

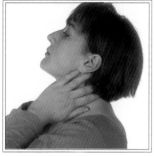

1 For stiff, aching neck muscles massage the neck with firm circular movements. Try to keep the arms relaxed.

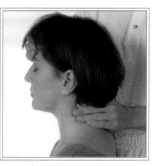

2 Ideally get someone else to massage the neck for you. They can also support your head while they massage.

NEURALGIA

Neuralgia is a sharp pain originating along the course of one or more nerves, and may come about from a variety of causes; both sciatica and shingles (see pages 26 and 27) give rise to forms of neuralgic pain. Facial neuralgia, affecting one of the trigeminal nerves in the face, can give intense pain, and may relate to stress, migraines or dental problems.

AROMATHERAPY

Using warm compresses (see page 15), including analgesic oils, over the affected areas can give much relief. Choose from Chamomile, Lavender, Marjoram or Rosemary oils – alternate the oil used for recurrent pains, or blend them together for greater effect.

HERBALISM

An infusion (see page 12) of Lavender (*Lavandula vera*) flowers, Lime Blossom (*Tilia europaea*) and Rosemary (*Rosmarinus officinalis*) leaves can be very helpful, not only to ease the pains but to ease tension and tone the nervous system. This mixture can also be used as a warm compress directly over the area.

Two other helpful herbs as infusions are:

ST JOHN'S WORT (*Hypericum perforatum*): anti-inflammatory and a nervous restorative. The blood-red oil made by infusing the flowers in pure vegetable oil

VERVAIN
(*Verbena officinalis*)

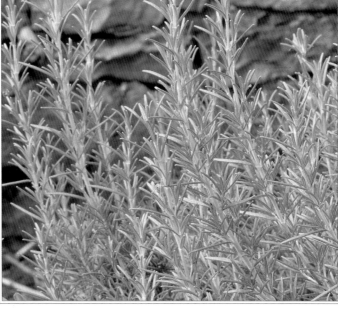

(see page 13) is an excellent local analgesic and healer.

VERVAIN (*Verbena officinalis*): a relaxant and nervous tonic, very helpful when neuralgia is related to being generally run-down and exhausted.

HOMEOPATHY

In the short term, try the following:
ACTAEA RAC: for facial neuralgia with pains into the cheekbone and as if piercing the eyeball. Pains ease at night.
BELLADONNA: for a hot, burning and flushed face, with mostly right-sided neuralgic pains and twitching muscles.

ROSEMARY (*Rosmarinus officinalis*)

GELSEMIUM: for pains radiating from the neck into the face, possibly with some nausea; migraine-related neuralgia.

NATUROPATHY

Simply using alternating hot and cold compresses, 3-4 minutes hot and a maximum 1 minute cold, repeated a few times, can ease the pains. For chronic sufferers a Vitamin B complex supplement can help to nourish the nervous system. In addition, look at ways of reducing stress such as relaxation or yoga classes.

SCIATICA

Pains along some point of the sciatic nerves, running from the low back down either leg to the foot, are a common form of neuralgia (see page 25). The pains may come about from an injury, and treatment from an osteopath or chiropractor should always be considered as one of the best ways to correct the cause. Poor posture, badly designed chairs or even a full back pocket can all cause pressure and pain in the sciatic nerve.

AROMATHERAPY

Initially, use cold compresses (see page 15) with either Chamomile or Lavender oils included. When the pains are less acute, or in longer-lasting sciatic discomfort, try warm compresses as suggested for Neuralgia (see page 25).

These oils are very helpful, diluted 2 per cent in a base oil and slowly massaged into the affected area.

HERBALISM

Chamomile *(Chamomilla recutita)* or Lavender *(Lavandula vera)* are also two useful herbs to take in infusion (see page 12) to ease muscle spasm and inflammation which add to the pains. For acute muscle spasms in the thigh or legs, try making a strong decoction (see page 12) of Cramp Bark (European Cranberry Bush) *(Viburnum opulus)* and using as a warm compress. A small cupful of this may be taken internally as a powerful relaxant.

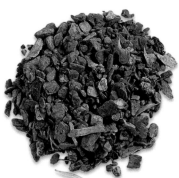

CRAMP BARK (EUROPEAN CRANBERRY BUSH)
(Viburnum opulus)

IMPROVING YOUR POSTURE

Apart from the suggestions listed on this page, you may want to consider help with improving your posture, learning how to move and hold yourself comfortably. The Alexander Technique and the Feldenkrais Technique are two systems that can help here; there are many qualified teachers of both available. Massage is not generally suitable in an acute phase, but in the longer term it is very helpful (see below for self-massage, or find a good massage therapist for best results).

HOMEOPATHY

ARSEN ALB: for intermittent pains shooting from the thigh down to the knee or even ankle.
IGNATIA: for sharp pains in the lower back and upper thighs, eased by walking around.
RHUS TOX: for severe pains in the hip, radiating down to the knee and causing limping. Generally these pains are worse in damp weather.

NATUROPATHY

Hot and cold compresses, as described for Neuralgia (see page 25), may give relief. Gentle exercise is generally useful, but stop if it becomes too painful. Take a serious look at your posture, how you bend, pick things up and so on. It is important to try to keep your back fairly upright, using your legs

---

LAVENDER
(Lavandula 'Nana')

to bend or to take the weight.

Look carefully at all the chairs you use. Sit well back on a chair, and use cushions if necessary to get you into a more comfortable position. In general, avoid staying in one position for too long, as the muscles begin to tighten and stiffen. For example, try to have regular breaks on a long car journey, or walk about for a while on the train.

To help ease sciatic pain, massage diluted essential oils, as recommended, into the buttock and upper thigh with slow circular movements.

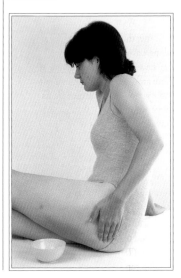

ASTHMA

Asthma is not generally a problem that should simply be tackled at home; it requires professional treatment and attention. Childhood asthma tends to be associated with an allergic response; there may also be hay fever and/or eczema present in the family. In trying to identify the allergens responsible it is often valuable to look further at external factors and also internal ones such as diet, as well as conventional skin testing.

AROMATHERAPY

During an actual attack of asthma, simply sniffing the aroma of a couple of drops of essential oil on a paper tissue may give relief from the spasm of the airways – choose from Lavender, Bergamot, Frankincense or Chamomile. In between attacks, massaging a choice of the above oils, diluted (see page 17), into the chest may help to prevent the spasms and build-up of thick mucus which gives the wheezing symptoms.

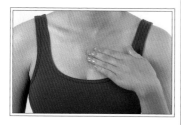

Essential oils, diluted in a base oil as recommended, can be massaged into the chest to relax the airways and ease breathing.

HERBALISM

Professional practitioners may use remedies which directly reduce the allergic response, or dilate the bronchial passageways, depending

CHAMOMILE
(Chamomilla recutita)

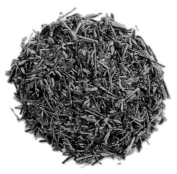

EYEBRIGHT *(Euphrasia officinalis)*

on specific individual needs. In between asthma attacks, taking an infusion (see page 12) of a mixture of Chamomile (*Chamomilla recutita*), Eyebright (*Euphrasia officinalis*) and Lavender (*Lavandula vera*) may help to relax the airways, tone up the mucous membranes and reduce inflammation and irritability of the bronchi.

HOMEOPATHY

The professional will similarly look to treat each person individually, so only consider the remedies below in the short term:

ACONITE: at the earliest sign of breathing problems, especially if brought on by a cold, or simply cold weather with strong winds, and where there is much anxiety or fear.

ARSENICUM: when symptoms are worse after midnight, with restlessness and a feeling of exhaustion.

IPECACUANHA: where there is wheezing, with a persistent, rattly cough accompanied by a strong feeling of nausea.

NATUROPATHY

For childhood asthma, or where there is a lot of thick mucus, it is well worth trying a change of diet, to exclude cows' milk products for a while, to decrease sugary baking products and sweets (candy), and to increase fresh vegetables and fruit.

Breathing exercises may be of help, especially for later-onset asthma or when exercise seems to aggravate the condition; a simple method of deepening the breathing pattern is to

A useful breathing exercise for asthma is simply to blow up a couple of balloons a day, to deepen the breath and exercise the diaphragm.

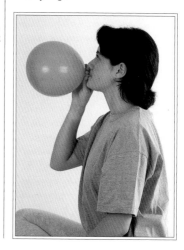

BREATHING EXERCISES

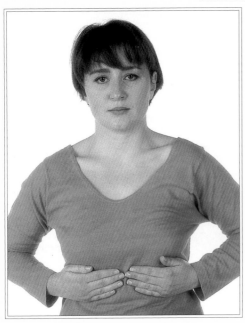

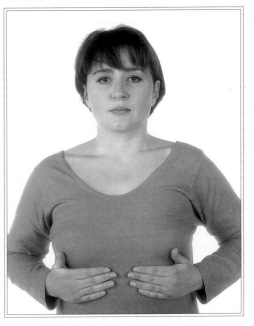

1 Place hands just below the breastbone and take a slow, deep breath. As you breathe in, push out the stomach; this should make the hands move apart a little, as the diaphragm moves.

2 As you breathe out, pull the stomach in. The diaphragm moves back up and the hands come together again. Repeat just 3 or 4 times and then breathe normally.

blow up balloons – for a maximum effect blow them up until they burst! Regular back massage will help release muscle tensions and improve circulation. Using hot and cold compresses (see page 15) on the upper back and/or chest will also stimulate circulation through the lungs and help remove mucus.

FRENCH LAVENDER
(*Lavandula stoechas*)

To stimulate circulation into the back and chest, and loosen phlegm in the lungs, place hands in a cupped shape on the upper back and briskly move them alternately up

and down. This should make a hollow sound on the back – slapping is not helpful, or enjoyable! (Be prepared for some coughing if the chest is congested.)

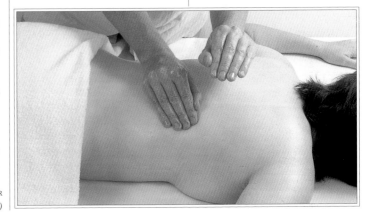

BRONCHITIS

Acute bronchitis, which typically follows an upper respiratory infection such as a heavy cold or influenza, produces a painful dry cough as the infected bronchi become inflamed. This leads to lots of mucus being produced and the cough becoming looser. The condition can recur, and chronic bronchitis is known as the "English disease" due to its frequent occurrence in England.

AROMATHERAPY

Essential oils, used primarily in steam inhalations (see below), are an excellent way to treat bronchitis. In the acute stage using powerfully antiseptic oils such as Lavender, Eucalyptus, Thyme or Tea Tree will be very useful. This can be backed up by gently rubbing a little diluted Lavender oil on to the chest – use 5 drops in 5ml (1 tsp) of olive oil or similar vegetable oil.

For more chronic symptoms choose from one of the following oils which are derived from gums or resins, or simply combine all three in an inhalation. BENZOIN: is most famous as the ingredient in Friar's Balsam; it has a warming and relaxing effect on the bronchi, and aids expectoration of the thick mucus.

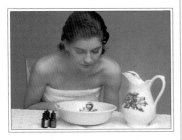

To make an inhalation, choose a bowl large enough to take at least 600 ml (1 pt/2½ cups) of water. Fill it with boiling water and add 2-3 drops of essential oil. As the oils vaporize, inhale the steam as deeply as possible. If you hold a towel over your head this will delay the effects of evaporation. Be careful to place the bowl in a safe position.

SELF-HELP MEASURES
There may not be any infection present in the chronic state; repeated irritation of the lungs produces excess mucus which clogs up the bronchi. Self-help measures include not smoking or being in smoky atmospheres, treating colds and so on promptly, not going out in foggy weather, and using steam inhalations to warm and moisten the airways.

FRANKINCENSE: another expectorant, which slows and deepens the breathing as well as being a good antiseptic agent. MYRRH: strongly anti-infective, helping to loosen the sticky mucus and shift it off the chest.

HERBALISM

There is a whole treasure chest of herbal medicines for different stages or states of bronchitis; if in doubt do seek professional advice. At the beginning, where there may be a feeling of chill, a tea from fresh Ginger (*Zingiber officinalis*) with perhaps a pinch of Cayenne pepper added will give warmth very quickly. Painful, harsh coughs can be soothed with infusions of Marshmallow leaf (*Althea officinalis*), Hyssop (*Hyssopus officinalis*) and Thyme (*Thymus vulgaris*), or else use White Horehound (*Marrubium vulgare*), an anti-spasmodic and expectorant remedy. A regular intake of garlic, ideally fresh, not only helps to stimulate the removal of excess mucus in chronic bronchitis, but is one of the most powerful anti-infective agents there is, helping to build resistance to all respiratory infections.

HOMEOPATHY

In the acute phase, look at these remedies, but seek qualified treatment if symptoms persist or chest pains set in.
ACONITE: for use in the early stages, with painful, dry cough and much restlessness, with a slight fever.
BRYONIA: for a dry, hacking cough which is made worse by changes in temperature, such as coming into a warm room.
IPECACUANHA: for a spasmodic cough with much rattly mucus on the chest, and a tendency towards vomiting.
PHOSPHORUS: for a hoarse voice, even going altogether, and a dry tickly cough, with a tight feeling like a band around the chest.

NATUROPATHY

Reduce mucus-forming foods: these are primarily dairy products, and also refined carbohydrates such as cakes and pastries. If the weather is damp or foggy, stay indoors, but also avoid rooms being too dry and hot. In chronic cases walking or other exercise in good weather will improve breathing. Hot and cold compresses (see page 15) will really stimulate circulation through the lungs and help breathing.

CATARRH

Irritation of the membranes of the nose and throat will encourage production of mucus; where this becomes excessive or prolonged, for example after a cold, then catarrh is the result. When this occurs lower down the airways, bronchial catarrh follows (see Bronchitis, page 33). Nasal catarrh is even more common in damp climates and the same advice is applicable.

AROMATHERAPY

Where there is a lot of nasal congestion, a steam inhalation with essential oils (see page 33) can be instantly effective in giving relief. In the short term Peppermint is excellent, especially combined with Eucalyptus and/or Tea Tree, to loosen thick, sticky mucus and fight any infection present. For longer term catarrhal problems, try using oil of Pine instead of Peppermint, perhaps with Chamomile, Lavender or Tea Tree.

HERBALISM

Apart from using steam inhalations for temporary relief, either with oils as described above or using a handful each of Peppermint (*Mentha piperita*) leaves, Eucalyptus (*Eucalyptus globulus*) leaves and Chamomile (*Chamomilla*

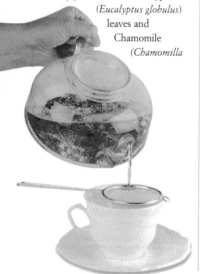

recutita) flowers to 1 litre (1¼ pt/4 cups) of boiling water, catarrh can often be very successfully treated with infusions (see page 12) of the following:
CATMINT (*Nepeta cataria*): helps to ease nasal congestion and improve the circulation through the nasal passages.
ELDERFLOWER (*Sambucus nigra*): has an anti-inflammatory effect, reducing swelling of the membranes and easing mucus production.
GOLDEN ROD (*Solidago virgaurea*): astringent, toning up the membranes and also reducing excess mucus.
HYSSOP (*Hyssopus officinalis*): loosens up thick phlegm, while calming the breathing; good if there is restlessness and problems with sleeping due to difficulty in breathing.

HOMEOPATHY

Initially think of one of these remedies:
ARSEN ALB: for running, watery catarrh, with a dripping nose.
HYDRASTIS: for a constant post-nasal drip, perhaps associated with blocked Eustachian tubes (connecting to the middle ear), creating a little deafness.
KALI BICH: where there is thick, stringy mucus, which is difficult to shift.
PULSATILLA: in chronic cases, where the catarrh varies at times from clear to a greenish-yellow colour.

Place 25 g (1 oz) dried Chamomile (Chamomilla recutita) *leaves in a teapot and pour on boiling water. Allow to infuse for 5 minutes. Strain and drink a cupful.*

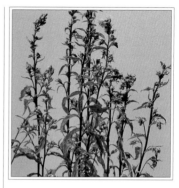

GOLDEN ROD (*Solidago virgaurea*)

NATUROPATHY

Avoid all mucus-forming foods, especially milk and other dairy products, and refined carbohydrates – most breakfasts of cereal and milk fall into this category, as do pastries, cakes and so on. Drinking warm fruit juices can often be helpful. If the catarrh tends to follow on from regular colds, a daily supplement of Vitamin C, up to 500 mg in strength, may need to be taken for a while.

Regular intake of garlic is invaluable in building up resistance to respiratory infections – ideally raw – and since the smell may stop other people coming near you, so colds are harder to catch! Actually, the smelly oil is the most anti-infective part of garlic, and 99 per cent of it is excreted out via the lungs so it works very strongly on the respiratory system. Odourless garlic perles, or capsules, will also work, although not as powerfully as the raw ingredient.

COLDS

Since there are over 200 strains of cold virus, it is not surprising that a cure has not been found. Prevention is better than treatment by far; once a cold has developed, it generally has to run its course. However, treatments can help to relieve symptoms and also stop the cold turning into persistent catarrh or a deeper infection.

AROMATHERAPY

Two methods are most appropriate for using oils to combat cold symptoms and stop complications: steam inhalations (see page 33) and baths. If, in the early stages, the cold is accompanied by a chill, adding 10 drops of Lavender and 5 drops of Cinnamon oil to a warm bath at night will help a lot. More stimulating oils such as Eucalyptus or Tea Tree (10 drops of each) can be used in baths earlier in the day. All the above are valuable in inhalations; a mixture often works better than just one oil.

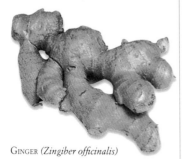

GINGER *(Zingiber officinalis)*

HERBALISM

One of the herbalists' most traditional standbys for colds is still one of the best: use an infusion (see page 12) of equal amounts of Peppermint *(Mentha piperita)*, Elderflower *(Sambucus nigra)* and Yarrow *(Achillea millefolium)*. Taken hot just before going to bed, this will induce a sweat, and if the cold is caught early enough, may stop it altogether. Even if too late for this, it will still be

very useful. Other herbs that may be added to the infusion include:
CAYENNE *(Capsicum minimum)*: a favourite North American Indian remedy: use 1.25 ml (¼ tsp) of the powder to really stimulate the circulation.
CINNAMON *(Cinnamomum zeylanicum)*: use a cinnamon stick, and break it into the mixture of herbs, for a gentle, warming and sweat-inducing effect.
GINGER *(Zingiber officinalis)*: grate a small piece of fresh root ginger into the mixture for extra heat.

HOMEOPATHY

ACONITE: for early stages of colds, when starting suddenly, perhaps after exposure to cold winds.
GELSEMIUM: for influenza-like symptoms, feeling chilly and trembling but with a flushed face.
NAT MUR: when there is a lot of sneezing, the nose is sore and inflamed and producing lots of mucus, either watery or like raw egg-white.

Fresh fruit is a natural source of Vitamin C.

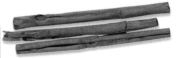

CINNAMON *(Cinnamomum zeylanicum)*

NATUROPATHY

Immediately increase Vitamin C intake; at the earliest stages very high doses of a Vitamin C supplement, up to 2,000 mg, may stop the infection alone, but if left too late, this is not needed and may make the bowels too loose. 500 mg is an ample dose to take regularly until the remaining symptoms clear up. Another useful supplement is sucking zinc lozenges, with up to 20 mg zinc gluconate in them, every 3-4 hours initially (taking *tablets* does not have the same effect).

Eat lots of fresh fruit for natural Vitamin A, B and C, and add plenty of raw garlic to food. Cut out sugary, starchy or milky foods. A short cleansing diet of just fresh fruit and salads, and plenty of liquids such as warm fruit juices or herb teas, will encourage the body to throw off the cold more effectively.

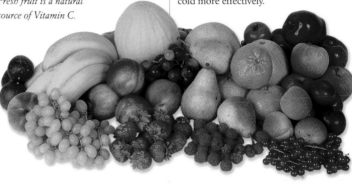

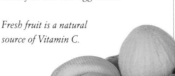

COUGHS

A cough is a natural reflex reaction to any irritation, inflammation or blockage in the airways. It often accompanies an infection such as a cold or bronchitis, but may come about through nervousness, with no direct irritation at all. By keeping the bronchial tubes open and clear, coughing can be of vital importance, and treatment should generally be aimed first at making the cough more effective rather than just suppressing it.

AROMATHERAPY

A useful way to help a cough do its job more effectively is by using oils in a steam inhalation (see page 33); oils can be chosen to soothe the lining of the air passages, fight infection if needed, and loosen mucus to make it easier to be removed.

Soothing oils include Benzoin and Lavender. Many essential oils are antiseptic, especially Thyme and Eucalyptus; to increase expectoration choose Frankincense or Marjoram. In fact all the above oils are helpful for tackling coughs. Choose a blend that you like the smell of – and remember that if the cough does not improve within a few days, seek professional help, especially for children.

THYME *(Thymus vulgaris)*

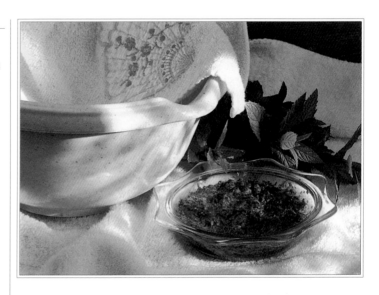

HERBALISM

This is an area where herbs are of special benefit; if in doubt get qualified treatment. Choose from one or a mixture of the following, taken as warm infusions (see page 12).

COLTSFOOT *(Tussilago farfara)*: one of the best cough remedies, particularly for irritating, spasmodic coughs. It will soothe, loosen mucus and reduce the spasm.

HYSSOP *(Hyssopus officinalis)*: a calming and relaxing expectorant, when the cough is

Fresh or dried herbs can be used to make a steam inhalation, to loosen congested mucus and open the airways.

associated with restlessness and irritation.

MARSHMALLOW *(Althea officinalis)*: a demulcent remedy, which means it is highly soothing to the inflamed tubes. For a harsh, dry and painful cough always include Marshmallow in a mixture, to ease the soreness.

THYME *(Thymus vulgaris)*: powerfully antiseptic, this relieves a dry cough linked with a respiratory infection.

WHITE HOREHOUND *(Marrubium vulgare)*: an expectorant, freeing up thick, sticky mucus and helping it to be removed more effectively.

TYPES OF COUGH
It can be useful to divide coughs
into two types; when the
membranes are hot and dry the
cough is painful and non-
productive. As mucus is produced,
the cough becomes moist, looser
and can feel almost choking. The
first kind needs soothing, while the
latter requires help in removing the
excess mucus. Choose the
appropriate treatments in each case.

HOMEOPATHY

For short-term treatment of a
cough, try a few doses (see page
10) of one of these remedies:
ACONITE: for a dry, short cough which
may occur first thing in the morning, or
come on after exposure to cold, dry
winds.
BRYONIA: for a really spasmodic, dry
cough which shakes the whole body
and is worse with movement or after
eating.
IPECACUANHA: for a moist cough, with
some wheezing and a feeling of
choking, and often much nausea.
PHOSPHORUS: for a dry, irritating and
tickly cough, made worse by changes in
temperature.

NATUROPATHY

Initially coughs are often quite
dry and painful; taking a little
honey from a spoon will help to soothe
this. To make the honey much more

powerful, try mashing a little chopped
raw onion or garlic into it first; it is anti-
social but very effective! Cut out all
dairy products from the diet, to reduce
the catarrh.
 Either steam inhalations or a hot
compress (see page 15) will encourage
expectoration and stimulate the lungs
to work better.
 Once a cough has been eased, try not
to slip back into eating patterns which
include a lot of sugar, dairy products,
cakes or pastries, as this can lower
resistance to infection and help the
cough to linger on or even to return in
full force.

Fields of commercially-grown lavender.

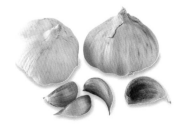

GARLIC *(Allium sativum)*

 For children, and for anybody where
the cause is unknown, when the cough
persists it is important to seek medical
advice, as professional help may be
needed. Similarly, if the mucus is bright
green or yellow this indicates the
presence of an infection, and advice
should be sought.

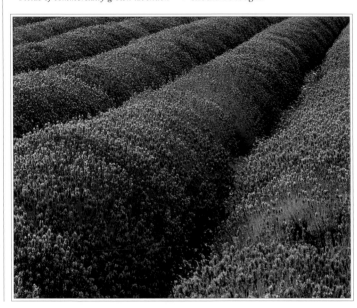

EARACHE

Earaches most often develop through an infection, perhaps following a cold or sinusitis, for instance. Because infections can spread through into the middle or even inner ear, with potentially serious complications, earaches should not be neglected. If an earache is associated with catarrh, this should be treated too. Do *not* put anything into the ear unless it has been examined to ensure that the eardrum is not perforated.

AROMATHERAPY

Use hot compresses (see page 15) over the ear to draw the inflammation outwards, and hopefully help any pus that may be present to come out also. Two very good oils to use are Chamomile and Lavender; a combination of both may be most effective.

HERBALISM

Hot compresses are the most effective home treatment; Chamomile *(Chamomilla recutita)* may be used as an infusion (see page 12) for this purpose too. Taking garlic internally will help to reduce any catarrh and fight infection – if on proper examination the eardrum is not perforated, then a clove of garlic can be crushed into 5 ml (1 tsp) of olive

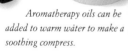

Aromatherapy oils can be added to warm water to make a soothing compress.

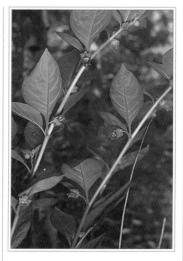

BELLADONNA *(Atropa belladonna)*

oil; this is warmed to blood temperature and a few drops gently inserted into the ear for an excellent local antibiotic.

HOMEOPATHY

As acute remedies only, choose from the following:
BELLADONNA: for throbbing pains, with a flushed face, a lot of heat around the ear and perhaps a high temperature.
HEPAR SULPH: for a very painful ear, very tender to touch, and which may be discharging offensive pus – this situation

---

EARACHE IN CHILDREN
Earaches, especially in children, need to be treated quickly as an infection within the middle ear can be both painful and damaging. Speedy home help can be very useful to avoid these problems, but get medical help if earache worsens or persists.

requires medical attention quite quickly so do not let it go on unchecked.
PULSATILLA: if there is a lot of thick, green catarrh present, and the earache and congestion is worse in hot rooms or stuffy atmospheres.

NATUROPATHY

Apart from all the local treatments by compress suggested above, follow the advice given for Catarrh (see page 34), especially if there is a pattern of recurring earaches, as prevention should be the primary aim.

CHAMOMILE *(Chamomilla recutita)*

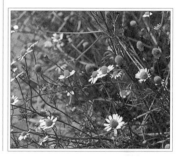

HAY FEVER

Hay fever is an allergic reaction, which can be triggered not just by grass pollens but in some people by various flower or tree pollens too. It is often seen together with other allergic reactions such as asthma and/or eczema, and if it is not relieved by the suggested self-help approaches, then seek qualified treatment. Practitioners may well start to act preventively before the hay fever season.

AROMATHERAPY

Simply sniffing a drop or two of an essential oil may be the best method; steam inhalations (see page 33) can be used but might be too hot for some people. You may well need to vary the oils used through the hay fever season, as they can become less effective if used for too long. Choose from Chamomile, Tea Tree, Pine, Melissa or Eucalyptus.

HERBALISM

Two herbs are very helpful in reducing the symptoms of hay fever: Chamomile (*Chamomilla recutita*) and Eyebright (*Euphrasia officinalis*).

Make an infusion of Chamomile (Chamomilla recutita), when cool soak a couple of cotton pads and place on the eyes. Rest for 10 minutes with the pads in place.

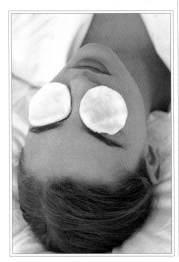

HAYFEVER SYMPTOMS

The membranes lining the nose are most often affected, with either congestion or else a streaming nose and sneezing; frequently the eyes or throat become inflamed too. An all-year-round allergic reaction, or allergic rhinitis, can be set up, with symptoms triggered by mould spores, house dust, fur and car exhaust fumes, for instance.

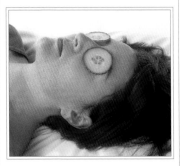

Slices of cucumber may be used on tired, sore eyes in the same way as herb pads.

They can both be used in two ways: firstly, as a tea taken 2 or 3 times a day (in severe cases try an infusion for stronger effect, see page 12) to reduce the inflammation and excess mucus, and, secondly, by soaking pads of cotton wool in a cooled infusion and placing on the eyelids to soothe sore, irritated eyes.

Where the mucus is very watery, alternative internal infusions to the above, or additions to them are:

GROUND IVY (*Glechoma hederacea*): very astringent, reducing excess mucus and drying out the secretions.

RIBWORT (*Plantago lanceolata*): also anti-catarrhal and astringent, toning up and healing the membranes.

HOMEOPATHY

Sometimes it can be worth using Mixed Pollens themselves in homeopathic dilution, before symptoms have started. Otherwise choose from:

ALLIUM CEPA: for a burning nasal discharge; the eyes will run too (think of your reaction to cutting up onions!).

ARSEN ALB: if the eyes are burning, with tears that feel hot. If the nose runs, that too will feel burning, sneezing gives no relief to the irritation.

EUPHRASIA: if the nose runs profusely, with lots of watery mucus, although it may block at night; the eyes feel sore and gritty, with burning tears.

NATUROPATHY

Reduce mucus production by cutting out dairy products (also see Catarrh, page 34), and when the symptoms are severe, take high levels of Vitamin C (up to 2,000 mg per day, unless diarrhoea occurs) to act as a natural anti-histamine.

Rinse out the eyes with an eyebath, using cool distilled water or a proprietary eyewash, to give temporary relief – you can also ease the nose by sniffing up distilled water to wash out the pollens.

INFLUENZA

Anyone who has had influenza will know that it is a more serious complaint than simply having a bad cold. Different viral strains produce differing symptoms, but generally there is a fever, aching muscles, headache and general weakness. Sometimes there may also be a harsh cough. In older, frail people it can seriously debilitate.

AROMATHERAPY

Several oils have considerable anti-viral activity, and help to boost the immune system. It is important though to use them at the earliest sign of influenza for maximum benefit. Either use them in the bath or as steam inhalations (see pages 8 and 33); it may also be a good idea to fumigate the house with oils at the same time, to help prevent everyone else getting the infection. This is best done by either putting 2-3 drops on a radiator to evaporate or else adding around 10 drops to a small plant spray filled with water, frequently spraying the room.

Dried herbs enable you to enjoy herbal teas all year long and are as effective as fresh herbs.

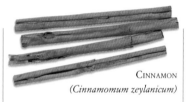

CINNAMON
(*Cinnamomum zeylanicum*)

Choose from Tea Tree, Eucalyptus, Lemon or Lavender oils.

HERBALISM

In the early stages of a chilled feeling, use a warming tea such as Cinnamon (*Cinnamomum zeylanicum*) – break a stick into a teapot – perhaps with 2.5 ml (½ tsp) of Cayenne (*Capsicum minimum*) or ground Ginger (*Zingiber officinalis*) added. When feeling more feverish, you can provoke sweating by taking infusions (see page 12) of Catmint (*Nepeta cataria*) and/or Elderflower (*Sambucus nigra*). The deep muscular aching can be relieved by using an infusion of Boneset (*Eupatorium perfoliatum*), either on its own or mixed with either of the above.

To stimulate the immune system, and also ward off complications such as bronchitis, take plenty of garlic, preferably raw – hot garlic bread or toast is a nice way to take it for all the family.

HOMEOPATHY

Choose from these remedies if not able to get professional treatment:
BRYONIA: if feeling very hot and dry, thirsty for cold drinks, aching all over, headache made worse by movement.

GELSEMIUM: for a hot head and face, but with chills that go up and down the back; burning headache but without any real sense of thirst.
NUX VOMICA: for thoroughly chilled feelings, cannot get warm at all, limbs and back are aching, stomach upset.

NATUROPATHY

At an early stage try having a hot bath to which you add 30–60 ml (2–4 tbsp) of Epsom Salts, then go straight to bed.

Generally restrict the diet, drinking fruit juices until the feverish period has passed, and then starting on fruit, vegetables and whole grains at first. If very hot and sweaty, try applying a cool compress to the chest and trunk.

Immediately the symptoms start, it is advisable to take high levels of Vitamin C to boost the immune system, around 3,000-4,000 mg to start with, reducing over 3-4 days to 500 mg until completely better.

INFLUENZA STRAINS

Influenza occurs in bouts of epidemic proportions, with periodic changes in the viral strains responsible. This makes vaccination programmes more difficult and less effective. Influenza can be a real killer, and attention to good health to prevent the onset of serious symptoms is essential, especially for older people in winter.

LARYNGITIS

Laryngitis is an acute inflammation of the larynx and vocal chords, leading to a very sore throat, hoarseness and even loss of voice. It may follow on from a cold or other infection, or be due to overstraining the voice by shouting, severe coughing or irritations such as smoke or dust.

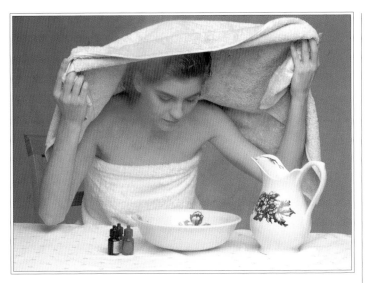

CAUSTICUM: for a hoarse voice, which may go completely, with a burning, raw throat and irritating cough.

PHOSPHORUS: if you cannot talk louder than a whisper, symptoms may have been brought on by overuse of the voice; with a dry cough and a desire for cold drinks and ice-cream.

NATUROPATHY

Cut out dairy produce to reduce excess catarrh, and take plenty of fruit juices. Try placing a cold compress (see page 15) around the throat, if the problem has been around for a while, it may be an idea to use a hot compress followed by a cold one. Sucking zinc gluconate lozenges not only soothes the throat but directly tackles any infection; in addition to fruit and juices it may be useful to take 500 mg of Vitamin C for a few days, or fresh lemon juice and honey drinks.

AROMATHERAPY

The best method for treatment is undoubtedly steam inhalation (see page 33); the natural choice of oil is probably Benzoin, but you could also use Sandalwood or Thyme. As the oils vaporize with the steam, they soothe the dry, inflamed membranes and ease the breathing as well as being highly antiseptic.

HERBALISM

Local treatment is by gargle; there are a number of useful herbs for this, they are most effective as tinctures (see page 14), otherwise use cooled infusions (see page 12). Choose from these astringent herbs: Sage (*Salvia officinalis*), Thyme (*Thymus vulgaris*), Agrimony (*Agrimonia eupatoria*) or

Holding a towel over your head will concentrate the herbal vapours and delay the effects of evaporation.

Raspberry Leaf (*Rubus idaeus*), which will help to tone up the puffy membranes. For a very soothing effect, add Marshmallow (*Althea officinalis*) to the gargle, or take 10 ml (2 tsp) of a decoction (see page 12) of the root 3 or 4 times a day.

HOMEOPATHY

One of these remedies should be suitable in the short term:
ACONITE: for sudden laryngitis following exposure to cold, dry winds, with a high temperature and a dry cough.

MARSHMALLOW
(*Althea officinalis*)

SINUSITIS

The sinus cavities are air spaces in the bones of the skull, behind, above and below the eyes. They act as a kind of sound-box, helping the voice to resonate. Like the nasal passages they are lined with mucous membranes, and an infection in the nose or throat can spread to the sinuses; acute sinusitis can be very painful and needs prompt treatment. Chronic sinusitis may be linked to allergic reactions such as hay fever.

AROMATHERAPY

Steam inhalations (see page 33) are the best way to work directly on the membranes, loosening thick mucus and fighting infection. Choose from oils of Chamomile, Eucalyptus, Lavender, Peppermint, Pine, Thyme or Tea Tree; a combination may be best, or else change around the oils. In acute sinusitis, the inhalations can be taken 4 times a day to ease the pain and relieve the congestion, reducing to once daily as the symptoms ease, until the sinuses have cleared up.

HERBALISM

Apart from steam inhalations as outlined above, using infusions internally (see page 12) can help to reduce the catarrh and inflammation. Look at the following herbs (see also Catarrh, page 34):

Oil of Eucalyptus is very effective used as part of a steam inhalation.

CATMINT *(Nepeta cataria)*: reduces nasal congestion and helps to liquefy the thick, sticky mucus.

ELDERFLOWER *(Sambucus nigra)*: reduces inflammation by improving circulation through the area, clears long-term catarrh, and eases congestion.

GOLDEN SEAL *(Hydrastis canadensis)*: has an astringent effect, cooling and toning up swollen, inflamed membranes. As this herb is quite expensive and difficult to find loose, it may be easier to take in tablet form, up to 500 mg a day.

It is also often very valuable to take plenty of garlic, either raw or as garlic perles, to fight any infection.

HOMEOPATHY

Try to match the remedy to the symptom pattern – look also at suggestions for Catarrh, Colds or Hay Fever (pages 34, 35 and 39).

CATMINT *(Nepeta cataria)*

HEPAR SULPH: for painful swelling of the nasal cavities, tender to the touch, with infected, yellow mucus discharge.

NAT MUR: a profuse, watery discharge, sneezing and a frontal headache are typical symptoms calling for this remedy.

SILICA: for a dry, blocked nose and a severe headache, perhaps with bouts of sneezing; worse with cold and better with warmth.

NATUROPATHY

Immediately cut out all dairy products, and restrict white flour, pastries, cakes and so on. Eat plenty of fresh fruit and vegetables. Avoid smoky atmospheres, and do not fly when nasal passages are acutely inflamed or blocked, as the changes in air pressure can given severe pain and could damage the eardrum.

Use alternating hot and cold light compresses (see page 15) or just splashes of water around the nose; start with hot water for about 3 minutes and then cold for no more than 1 minute, repeating 2 or 3 times. This will reduce congestion and inflammation, and thus ease the pains. Using an inhalation can be a helpful back-up to this.

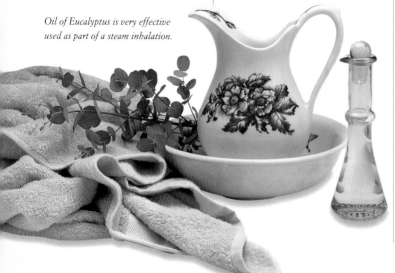

SORE THROATS

Sore throats are more and more common nowadays, with increased airborne pollution, smoky, dry atmospheres in air-conditioned buildings and so on. The irritation can range from an annoying tickle to a rasping soreness, and may be linked to other infections. Where the throat inflammation, or pharyngitis, also extends down to the larynx, the voice may be affected – see also Laryngitis and Tonsillitis (pages 41 and 44).

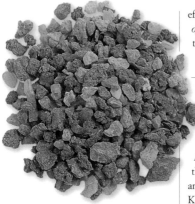

MYRRH *(Commiphora molmol)*

AROMATHERAPY

Use steam inhalations (see page 33) with oils such as Benzoin, Lavender or Thyme. One drop *only* of essential oil of Lemon on 2.5 ml (½ tsp) of honey acts as a powerful local antiseptic, as well as being soothing.

HERBALISM

If possible, use the following herbs as tinctures for gargling; if unavailable then use cooled infusions (see page 12): Agrimony *(Agrimonia eupatoria)*, Sage *(Salvia officinalis)*, and Thyme *(Thymus vulgaris)* are all astringent, toning up the membranes, the latter two also being quite antiseptic. For a more powerful effect try using a tincture (see page 14) of Myrrh *(Commiphora molmol)*, together with one or more of the others. If making infusions, add two broken liquorice sticks to give a more soothing

effect, or else use Marshmallow *(Althea officinalis)* leaf in equal amounts with the other herb(s).

HOMEOPATHY

The choice is wide, depending on the causes and the nature of the symptoms. It is advisable to look at other headings in this section too.

APIS MEL: for a red, swollen, burning throat and difficulty in swallowing anything.

KALI BICH: for sharp pains, relieved by swallowing, although there may also be a feeling of a "frog-in-the-throat" which is not relieved. The throat is especially dry and sore first thing in the mornings, with some sticky mucus.

MERC SOL: for a painful and raw throat, with a lot of watery, possibly unpleasant-smelling saliva.

NATUROPATHY

For adults and older children the diet can be restricted to fruit juices only for a day or two at most; younger children and infants will be unlikely to cope with this, so simply reduce the dairy foods and give plenty of fruit juices. If the throat is swollen and feels very hot, try a cold compress (see page 15) around it. If

AGRIMONY
(Agrimonia eupatoria)

OCCUPATIONAL HAZARDS

Many occupations involve excessive use of the voice e.g. teaching, and sore throats are commonplace. The regular use of herbal gargles can ease this discomfort, and help to prevent loss of voice or an actual infection. Keeping the throat moist by drinking liquids often, helps too.

---

available, suck zinc lozenges. Rest the voice and keep in a warm atmosphere.

In modern offices the dry air leads to frequent sore throats. Sip liquids often, and try to make the air more moist if possible, for example with plants.

SAGE *(Salvia officinalis)*

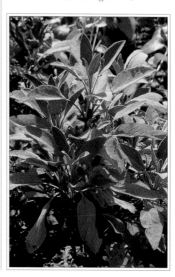

TONSILLITIS

I nflammation and infection of the tonsils most often occurs in children or younger adults;
it used to be the fashion to remove the tonsils but unless they become chronically badly
infected and act as a focus for other infections, it is now considered better to keep them.
They act as an early warning sign of lowered vitality, and if this first line of defence is lost,
then more deep-seated conditions can occur in later life.

AROMATHERAPY

Essential oils are not for internal use,
unless under qualified treatment, and
are rather unpleasant for local treatment.
In tonsillitis they are best used as
supportive treatment, using steam
inhalations (see page 33) of Benzoin,
Eucalyptus or Thyme to ease
inflammation and fight general infection.

HERBALISM

All the herbs mentioned under
Sore Throats (see page 43) for
gargling are excellent here too,
especially Myrrh (Commiphora
molmol), Thyme (Thymus vulgaris) and
Sage (Salvia officinalis). For repeated
bouts of tonsillitis take garlic daily,
either perles/capsules or fresh. Another
essential herb to use for chronic

GARLIC (Allium sativum)

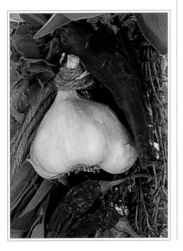

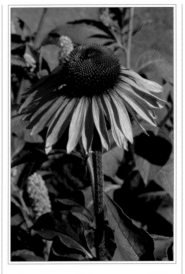

CONE FLOWER (Echinacea angustifolia)

tonsillitis is Cone Flower (Echinacea
angustifolia or E. purpurea); this boosts
the immune system and may be taken in
tablets or else as a tincture (see page
14), 20 drops twice daily.

HOMEOPATHY

Remedies applicable to tonsillitis
include:
ACONITE: for sudden onset of
inflammation, with hot, red and
burning tonsils and thirst for cold
drinks.
HEPAR SULPH: for pain on swallowing, as
if something is stuck in the throat, tonsils
swollen and discharging a yellow pus.
LYCOPODIUM: for chronic swelling of the
tonsils, which look as if they are pitted

with small white discharging ulcers;
cold drinks make the sensation worse.

NATUROPATHY

The tonsils' actions, in trapping
and removing infective bacteria
that would otherwise cause deeper
problems, means that they are more
easily infected themselves. This can
produce an infection of the adenoids
too, with nasal congestion.

Where these symptoms occur, it is
helpful to cut out dairy projects for a
while. In any case, take plenty of fluids,
especially fruit juices. Freshly-squeezed
lemon juice, with a little honey, is a
local antiseptic. Repeated attacks of
tonsillitis are often a sign of lowered
health in general, and may need
professional treatment.

THYME (Thymus vulgaris)

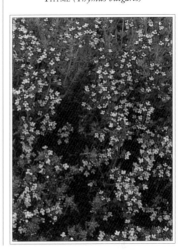

WHOOPING COUGH

This highly infectious bacterial infection tends to occur in epidemics every few years. Thick, sticky mucus gives rise to a spasmodic cough and the difficulty in inhaling with this gives the characteristic whooping sound. It is mostly seen in children, and in babies it can be serious, so get professional help as soon as possible. Symptoms can linger on for several weeks, so continue to help breathing by the measures listed below.

AROMATHERAPY

Relief for the condition is most dramatic with steam; either use inhalations (see page 33) or with infants simply hold them near steam, such as a basin filled with piping hot water or near a hot bath (make sure they do not touch very hot water). Very good oils to add to the steam are Cypress, Lavender and Tea Tree.

HERBALISM

Start to give herbal teas/infusions at the first sign of coughing – do not wait for the respiratory distress that can set in with the whoop. Use steam to free the mucus, as mentioned above. In young infants and babies, diluted teas

Keep all medicines and aromatherapy oils out of the reach of small children.

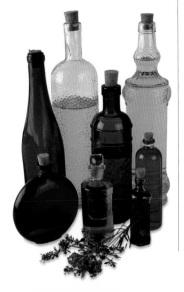

should be strong enough; older children may need infusions (see page 12), again diluted (for dosages see page 9). Look at these herbs, and use a blend of the most appropriate:
CHAMOMILE (*Chamomilla recutita*): helps to calm the person down, reduces catarrh and accompanying nausea.
COLTSFOOT (*Tussilago farfara*): one of the best cough remedies, helping to ease the spasmodic nature of the cough.
LAVENDER (*Lavandula vera*): a relaxing expectorant, soothing the cough and breathing and also generally calming.
THYME (*Thymus vulgaris*): highly antiseptic, soothing the dry cough that may herald the start of the problem.
WHITE HOREHOUND (*Marrubium vulgare*): good expectorant, loosening the sticky mucus and reducing spasm.

An alternative treatment that can work wonders is to chop or crush two cloves of garlic into 15 ml (1 tbsp) of honey and leave for a couple of hours, or even overnight. Give up to 5 ml (1 tsp) either neat or diluted in a little warm water, 4 times a day.

HOMEOPATHY

Ideally seek qualified advice for this ailment, but a remedy often used for the characteristic rapid paroxysmal cough is Drosera. Often the bout of coughing can result in vomiting. If children have been in contact with whooping cough, it can be worth trying this remedy as a prophylactic: give 3 doses of 30c dilution (see page 10) in a 24-hour period.

SELF-HELP MEASURES

Anyone who has heard the distinctive whooping sound will always remember whooping cough. Early treatment is most helpful; self-help measures such as steam treatments can speedily relieve symptoms, but babies and tiny infants should ideally be professionally checked as well.

NATUROPATHY

Keep the fluid intake high, especially if there is vomiting with the coughing bouts; also give only small amounts of light food rather than big meals. Avoid dairy products in order to lessen mucus production, and give easily digested foods.

For older children, supplementing diet with 500 mg Vitamin C daily for a couple of weeks will help to boost the immune system – reduce or stop if diarrhoea develops.

Try to keep the diet light, wholesome and low in dairy foods for quite a while after the initial symptoms have eased, as any build-up in mucus can cause more problems for several weeks.

WHITE HOREHOUND
(*Marrubium vulgare*)

THE CIRCULATORY SYSTEM

⊹⊱═◉ ◦ ◖═⊰⊹

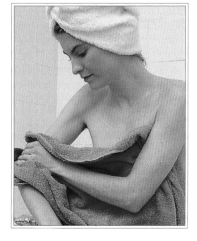

Cirrculation is absolutely vital for health; the blood transports oxygen and all our other nutrients around the body to all the cells, and carries away the waste materials from cellular activity. Without good circulation we simply do not have the fuel to provide enough energy for health. In cooler climates many people suffer from poor circulation, and lowered immune systems can often follow.

Disorders of circulation can occur in the heart or in the blood vessels; the former are not suitable for self-treatment, and for any prolonged or serious circulatory problems it is best to get professional treatment. For example, angina is a cramping of the heart muscles due to narrowing or obstruction of the coronary arteries. When the supply of oxygen to the cardiac muscles does not meet any extra demand, perhaps when walking uphill, the characteristic cramp and pains of angina occur for a short while. Resting eases the pain after a few minutes. Angina can be relieved by taking infusions of Lime Blossom *(Tilia europaea)*, but full professional treatment needs to look at individual causes as well as the health of the heart.

ABOVE: Alternating hot and cold baths is a useful self-help measure for improving circulation. Herbs such as Marigold (Calendula officinalis) (above left) and Witch Hazel (Hamamelis virginiana) can also help astringe and tone swollen veins.

CHILBLAINS

For people with poor peripheral circulation, living in cool, damp climates often creates chilblains. When circulation is reduced in cold weather, the oxygen supply to the fingers and toes is restricted to the point that the skin cells are damaged and swelling, redness and itching occurs. Warmer weather improves the condition, but using radiant heat, such as warming by the fire, can tend to aggravate the swelling and burning itchy sensation.

AROMATHERAPY

Only use oils locally if the skin is unbroken; otherwise an inflamed reaction may be set off. Massage the affected areas with warming oils such as Black Pepper, Ginger or Marjoram, using a vegetable oil containing a maximum of 3 per cent essential oil. For longer term treatment during the winter months, add oils of Cypress, Juniper, Pine or Rosemary to baths (see page 8 for dilutions), or use them diluted in a base oil as above for regular brisk massage of the hands and feet.

HERBALISM

Locally, use a footbath to which is added a decoction (see page 12) of fresh Ginger root (*Zingiber officinalis*), using up to 15 g (½ oz) per 750 ml (1¼ pt/ 2⅔ cups) of water, or add a tea made from ground Ginger, or for maximum circulatory-stimulating effect Cayenne (*Capsicum minimum*). Do not use the latter if the skin is broken.

Handbaths, or footbaths, are good ways to improve circulation to the extremities. Place hands in a bowl of hot water, with essential oils added as recommended.

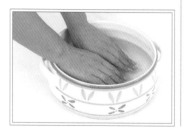

GINGER DECOCTION

Ginger can be made into a tea, but a stronger medicine is made from a decoction.

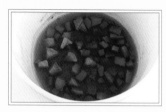

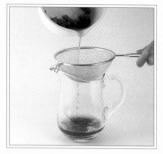

1 Simmer 15 g (½ oz) chopped rhizome in 750ml (1¼ pt/2⅔ cups) water until the liquid is reduced to about 600 ml (1 pt/2½ cups).

2 Strain through a sieve and store in a jug. Give in doses of 5-20 ml (1 tsp -1½ tbsp), three times a day. It will keep in the fridge for 3 days.

Internally, teas from the above herbs will generally improve circulation. For a gentler effect on the extremities use an infusion (see page 12) of Yarrow (*Achillea millefolium*); this dilates the tiny blood vessels in the hands and feet, helping them to warm.

HOMEOPATHY

Since treatment may be needed for a couple of weeks or so, use low potencies such as 6c (see page 10). AGARICUS: if the symptoms are worse when cold, and there is itching and burning with redness of the skin. CALCAREA CARBONICA: if there is relief from cold, the feet in particular feeling damp and cold to the touch. PETROLEUM: if, as well as burning and itching, there is chapping and cracking of the skin; typically the fingers get splits at the tips.

NATUROPATHY

Use alternating hot and cold foot or handbaths, using warm rather than too hot water, for about 4 minutes, and then cold for up to 1 minute. Make sure the feet or hands are well dried. Repeat for 10-15 minutes, nightly for a week if needed. Giving the hands or feet a brisk friction-rub daily will also help the circulation

Increase Vitamin C in the diet by eating more fresh fruit and potatoes; if you suffer badly from chilblains, take a supplement of Vitamin C, up to 1 mg until better, possibly together with 300–400 iu of Vitamin E to improve the elasticity of the blood vessels.

FEVER

The raising of the body temperature, usually in response to an infection, is something that natural medicine sees as generally a positive healing attempt by the body. Most of our vital processes are stimulated by the higher temperature, and conversely many infective organisms cannot survive as well, so the fever response is one that can be aided rather than instantly suppressed.

AROMATHERAPY

In order to encourage sweating at the stage of resolving the fever, a warm bath with a maximum of 10 drops of one of these oils may help – if bathing is not appropriate, use them at 1 per cent dilution in a little vegetable oil and massage the back or chest. Chamomile, Cypress, Lavender or Tea Tree are good choices. For a more cooling effect use 5 drops of oils of Eucalyptus, Lavender or Peppermint in a small bowl of tepid water and sponge the upper back, neck and chest.

HERBALISM

If at the early, shivery stage of an infection, use a tea with Ginger (*Zingiber officinalis*) – 2.5 ml (½ tsp) ground ginger, or peel and grate a small piece of fresh root – and Cinnamon (*Cinnamomum zeylanicum*) – 2.5 ml

CATMINT (*Nepeta cataria*)

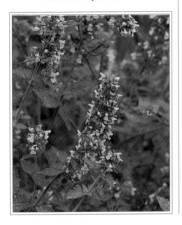

CHECKING THE TEMPERATURE
By taking the temperature, and checking on feelings of heat or cold, the stages of the fever can be noted and treatment given. Initially, our internal thermostat is turned up, making us feel cold and shivery; as circulation is boosted and we reach the higher levels, we can feel more comfortable, although with a raised temperature. If the process goes too high, or the infection is not controlled, the thermostat is reset back to normal and we feel feverish and hot. Sweating reduces the temperature. Body temperatures around 38°C (100-101°F) often give the best results in fighting infection. Children's temperatures often go higher, and so may an adult's; if left for too long this can make us feel very unwell and cooling may then be needed, either by inducing sweating or through sponging with tepid water. If in doubt get professional help.

(½ tsp) ground cinnamon, or half a cinnamon stick.

When the fever makes you hot and restless, sweating can be provoked by taking a hot infusion (see page 12) of Elderflower (*Sambucus nigra*). (At normal temperatures this will not make you sweat.) Other suitable infusions to

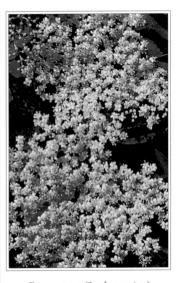

ELDERFLOWER (*Sambucus nigra*)

relieve the symptoms are: Boneset (*Eupatorium perfoliatum*), Catmint (*Nepeta cataria*), Peppermint (*Mentha piperita*) and Yarrow (*Achillea millefolium*), while Lime Blossom (*Tilia europaea*) can be added to aid the dilation of the blood vessels and assist general relaxation. Hyssop (*Hyssopus officinalis*) is another excellent herb to calm the system; a tea may be taken frequently while symptoms prevail.

HOMEOPATHY

As with herbalism, there are many homeopathic remedies available and the cause/exact reaction needs to be sorted out first. A few to choose from, in mild feverish states are:

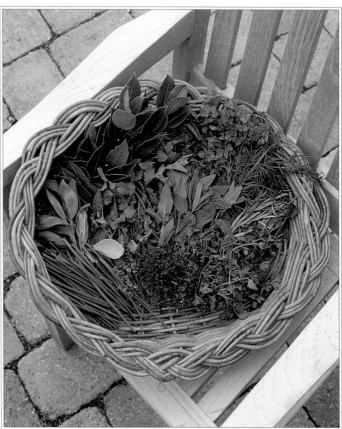

ACONITE: for dry, burning skin and great restlessness and agitation; symptoms may come on quickly.

BELLADONNA: for a high temperature, with a hot, very red face and a racing pulse. In extreme fever cases the person may also be delirious and highly excitable.

EUPATORIUM PERFOLIATUM: for an influenza-type of fever, with chills followed on by heat, aching muscles and maybe sweating.

FERRUM PHOS: for milder fevers, with less obvious causes; a hot, throbbing head and frequent sweating.

NATUROPATHY

Avoid active exercise; take plenty of rest but do not swaddle in heavy bedclothes; keep the room aired.

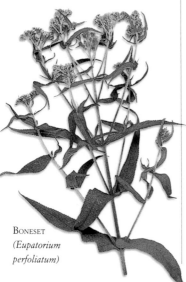

BONESET
(*Eupatorium perfoliatum*)

Herbs can help combat a fever by either provoking sweating, or by aiding the dilation of the blood vessels.

Drink fruit juices, herb teas or water, and restrict food until the temperature has returned to normal. Sponge the face and chest with tepid water if the temperature is too hot. A cold pack or compress around the trunk will also reduce excessive heat; use something large like a towel wrung out in cold water and wrapped around the body and then wrap in a larger, dry towel or blanket.

Feverish conditions used to be much more common, and traditional practitioners such as herbalists developed quite sophisticated techniques to deal with them. They have become rarer nowadays, but natural measures remain very important in helping to cope with a fever. If the temperature rises to the point where someone becomes delirious or even has a convulsion, get urgent medical aid. Young children can be quite prone to convulsions, but this is rarer as we get older.

HYSSOP
(*Hyssopus officinalis*)

HAEMORRHOIDS

Haemorrhoids, or piles, are swollen veins in the rectum due to a restricted local blood supply and congestion in the pelvic cavity. Occasionally they may protrude externally, and can give rise to bleeding especially with a bowel movement. Piles can occur during pregnancy due to the increased pressure, but are often associated with chronic constipation, when frequent straining to empty the bowels causes extra pressure on the veins.

AROMATHERAPY

Using oils such as Cypress or Juniper in the bath can help to stimulate pelvic circulation; also adding a couple of drops of either to a bowl of cool water and then using this for a compress (see page 15) may help too. Massage of the abdomen (see right) with a 2 per cent dilution of oils of Marjoram or Rosemary can help ease constipation and relieve haemorrhoids.

PILEWORT *(Ranunculus ficaria)*

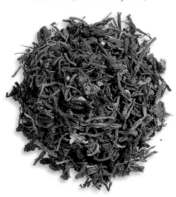

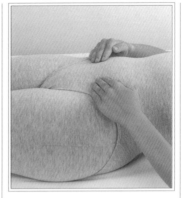

Press fingers steadily into the low abdomen, and massage with small circular movements, to release tension and improve local circulation.

to a small bowl of warm water.

Prolong bleeding from piles can eventually lead to anaemia. Drinking Nettle *(Urtica dioica)* tea may relieve this, but take steps to avoid constipation too.

HOMEOPATHY

Some possible remedies are:
AESCULUS: for a dry itching and stinging sensation, and a tendency for the veins to prolapse and protrude externally.
HAMAMELIS: for a burning soreness, often with bleeding.
SULPHUR: for hot, burning and itching in the anus; the pains are made worse by standing and better when lying.

NATUROPATHY

Practitioners in all of the therapies are likely to give dietary advice, and it is sensible to ensure you eat plenty of fresh vegetables and fruit to give adequate fibre and ease constipation, see also Constipation (page 57). Hot and cold compresses or even hot/cold baths will improve local circulation and reduce congestion; ice packs may be useful to reduce swelling at times. Exercise is also helpful to get the circulation going; ideally get individual advice. Avoid long periods of standing.

WITCH HAZEL
(Hamamelis virginiana)

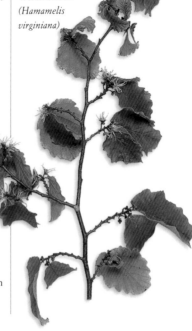

HERBALISM

Local treatment can help to astringe and tone the swollen veins. Use commercial creams made with extract of Pilewort *(Ranunculus ficaria)*, Horse Chestnut *(Aesculus hippocastanum)* or Marigold *(Calendula officinalis)*, or use a compress of distilled Witch Hazel *(Hamamelis virginiana)*; the tincture (see page 14) is much more astringent, if available use this diluted at the rate of 15 ml (1 tbsp)

POOR CIRCULATION

Poor circulation to the extremities is quite common in cooler climates, and particularly in elderly people or those who do very little exercise. (See also Chilblains, page 47). Poor circulation can lead on to more serious conditions such as phlebitis or thrombosis, so it should not be neglected, and professional medical help should be sought if in any doubt.

HAND MASSAGE

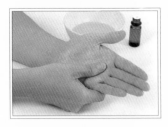

1 Place some base oil in a bowl, with essential oils added as recommended. Massage into palms of hands with a steady circular movement.

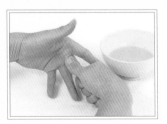

2 Squeeze down the fingers to stretch and loosen them, pushing towards the palm. Repeat steps 1 and 2 several times.

FOOT MASSAGE

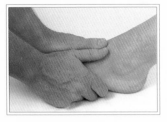

1 To stretch the feet, place hands with thumbs on top of the foot, keeping a firm grip with both of the hands.

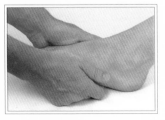

2 Move thumbs outward, as if breaking a piece of bread (be gentle with your partner!); repeat movement several times.

too, and cayenne pepper is the strongest circulatory stimulant, perhaps simply use in cooking for this effect as well as its flavour.

HOMEOPATHY

To improve circulation, the following remedies may be of help in the short term, but if symptoms persist and the fingers and toes become numb, then seek professional medical advice:

SECALE: For cold hands and feet with a burning sensation. The rest of the body also feels cold, and the fingers and

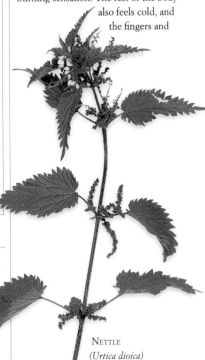

NETTLE
(*Urtica dioica*)

AROMATHERAPY

Massage the hands or feet with diluted oils such as Black Pepper, Lavender, Marjoram or Rosemary. These can be added to a warm footbath for a stronger short-term treatment. Use a maximum of 10 drops in total, and try a blend of 2 or 3 of these oils. Avoid if skin is broken, get advice first.

HERBALISM

Take hot herbal teas regularly to aid peripheral circulation; choose from Elderflower (*Sambucus nigra*), Ginger (*Zingiber officinalis*), Lime Blossom (*Tilia europaea*), Nettle (*Urtica dioica*) or Yarrow (*Achillea millefolium*). Daily intake of garlic stimulates blood flow

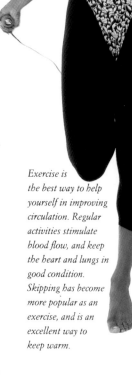

THE BLOODSTREAM

Since the circulation transports nourishment, both oxygen and nutrients from food, around the body it is essential for our overall health and vitality. Waste matter from all our cells is carried away in the bloodstream for elimination, and white blood cells form an essential part of our immune system. Keeping circulation flowing well, therefore, should be a priority for everyone.

As we get older, circulation tends to slow down and this is exaggerated if we stop exercising or being active. With increasingly sedentary lifestyles in many countries, it is very important to move as much as possible at work, or in retirement, to combat reduced circulation.

Exercise is the best way to help yourself in improving circulation. Regular activities stimulate blood flow, and keep the heart and lungs in good condition. Skipping has become more popular as an exercise, and is an excellent way to keep warm.

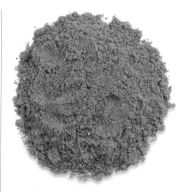

CAYENNE *(Capsicum minimum)*

with prominent veins. Skin can also appear blotchy.

toes can become quite blue or white. Take 6c every 30 minutes for up to 10 doses.
CARBO VEG: For cold hands and feet with a mottling of the skin. The skin feels icy cold to the touch and appears blue,

YARROW *(Achillea millefolium)*

NATUROPATHY

Various substances constrict the peripheral blood vessels, most notably caffeine and nicotine, so reducing or cutting out coffee and tobacco will help greatly. Exercise is another essential, wherever possible, and in colder weather keep the wrists and ankles warm as well as the hands and feet themselves. Additional amounts of Vitamin C (up to 500 mg per day) and Vitamin E (up to 400 iu per day) can boost circulation and aid the elasticity of the blood-vessel walls.

CAUTION
Do not increase the doses from those suggested here: it is likely to do more harm than good.

INDIGESTION

Indigestion is a general term for discomfort, often accompanied by bloating, acidity, heartburn, nausea or bowel disturbances (see other entries in this section). Usually it is a temporary problem, brought about by eating too much or the wrong kind of food, excess alcohol or from stress. Longer-term digestive pains may be caused among other reasons by taking aspirin-related drugs, by heavy smoking or other digestive ailments.

AROMATHERAPY

A warm compress (see page 15) including Chamomile or Lavender oils may give some relief, or try gently massaging a 2 per cent dilution of one of them into the abdomen if indigestion is milder.

HERBALISM

Herbal teas in the first place may well sort out the immediate indigestion, choose from:
CHAMOMILE (*Chamomilla recutita*): for the effects of over-eating, also if in a stressed state.
LEMON BALM (*Melissa officinalis*): for nervous indigestion; related to meals or not, settles a churning stomach.
MEADOWSWEET (*Filipendula ulmaria*): for acid indigestion, especially if accompanied by some looseness in the bowels.

LEMON BALM (*Melissa officinalis*)

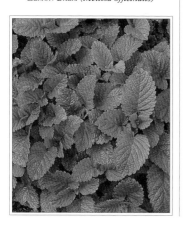

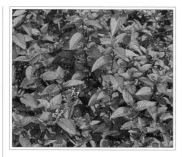

PEPPERMINT (*Mentha piperita*)

PEPPERMINT (*Mentha piperita*): for indigestion with plenty of flatulence and bloated abdomen, or even nausea. Also think of taking Slippery Elm (*Ulmus fulva*) if indigestion pains are persistent, either 5 ml (1 tsp) of the powder blended in a cupful of water, or the pure tablets, with one or more meals, to soothe the stomach.

HOMEOPATHY

For an occasional bout of indigestion, try a couple of doses (see page 10) of:
ARGENT NIT: where there is a lot of wind, with belching and possibly heartburn, a craving for sweet or fatty foods which tend to upset the digestion and give diarrhoea.
LYCOPODIUM: for pains and wind; if hungry but can only take small amounts of food, worse with cold foods or drink.
NUX VOMICA: useful for the effects of eating and drinking too much, causing pain, heartburn and even vomiting.

NATUROPATHY

If indigestion is quite bad, cut out solid food for 24 hours if possible, taking only herb teas or fruit juices (particularly pineapple which contains digestive enzymes), and reintroduce foods gently, starting with something light like soup or puréed apple. If indigestion is repetitive, try taking a Vitamin B complex supplement as a digestive stimulant, or else look at a digestive enzyme supplement such as Pepsin in the short term, but it may be better to get professional treatment. Avoid drinking lots of fluid at mealtimes, as this will dilute your natural digestive juices.

Chamomile tea is a relaxing aid to the digestive system.

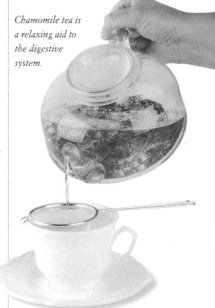

MOUTH ULCERS

These small ulcers, that can occur on the tongue, gums or the lining of the mouth, are sometimes due to local trauma, for instance biting your cheek or wearing ill-fitting dentures, but often they reflect a state of generally being run-down. Recurrent "crops" of mouth ulcers may therefore need more overall treatment; see Stress (pages 28-9) as well as anything directed locally.

AROMATHERAPY

The essential oil of choice for treating mouth ulcers is undoubtedly Myrrh. This is not only astringent and healing but also has an anti-fungal property; one of the reasons for mouth ulcers can be fungal infection, for example *Candida albicans* (the cause of thrush). Myrrh is best used in tincture form (see Herbalism below); you can make your own in small amounts by dissolving the essential oil in alcohol – use 5 drops in 5 ml (1 tsp) of a spirit such as vodka or brandy. This can be applied neat right on to the ulcers, or use 2.5 ml (½ tsp) in a little water as a mouthwash. You can add 1 drop of oil of Fennel to make it taste better, dissolving it thoroughly.

HERBALISM

Local treatment is by means of herbal tinctures (see page 14), to stimulate healing

and reduce the inflammation. The strongest, although worst tasting, is Myrrh (*Commiphora molmol*); others to choose from are Marigold (*Calendula officinalis*), Sage (*Salvia officinalis*) and Thyme (*Thymus vulgaris*). Pay attention to general health, and seek professional treatment if the ulcers are persistent or recurring. Cone Flower (*Echinacea angustifolia* or *E. purpurea*) may be a useful herb to take; it boosts the immune system and is widely obtainable in tablet form, or a tincture of the fresh plant is also available – take 10 drops in water 3 times a day.

HOMEOPATHY

Remedies are more likely to be of benefit if they are chosen for the background causes, but some examples of those remedies that are of value for the ulcers are:
BORAX: for painful small ulcers that feel hot in the mouth and may even bleed, when eating for instance.
MERC SOL: when there is an unpleasant, metallic taste in the mouth, with larger, almost greyish ulcers and perhaps bleeding gums; good for oral thrush.
NAT SULPH: for very painfully sensitive ulcers which may look like blisters, the discomfort is relieved by something cold such as an ice cube.

NATUROPATHY

Recurrent mouth ulcers can often indicate a poor diet, or nutritional deficiencies. Nutrients most likely to be

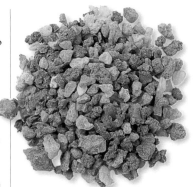

MYRRH (*Commiphora molmol*)

lacking, and consequently of most benefit in treating the problem, are Vitamin B2, Vitamin C and zinc, and supplements of these may be needed in the short term until the diet can be improved to give sufficient amounts – increase green leafy vegetables, fresh fruit, whole grain bread (including the wheatgerm) and for non-vegetarians eat some meat and fish.

Mouth ulcers most often occur at times of stress or when the immune system is lowered in some way, so it is generally advisable to look at ways of reducing the impact of stress (see pages 28-9) if ulcers are recurring frequently.

For direct local treatment, try applying pure wheatgerm oil, for example by piercing a natural, oil-based Vitamin E capsule, and dabbing a little on to the ulcer. If there are foods, for instance vinegar, that do aggravate the ulcers, obviously leave them out of the diet for a while.

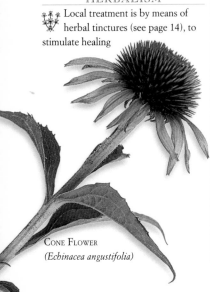

CONE FLOWER
(*Echinacea angustifolia*)

PRE-MENSTRUAL SYMPTOMS

There are a number of symptoms that can occur in the second half of the menstrual cycle, i.e. leading up to the period, due mostly to imbalances in hormone production. These symptoms tend to be lumped together by the medical profession into pre-menstrual syndrome (PMS), but not all women experience them in the same combination or in the same way.

AROMATHERAPY

Essential oils can be helpful in reducing fluid retention; this is most effectively done by using them with lymphatic drainage massage, so do see a professional aromatherapist if this is a major part of your symptoms. Using oils such as Geranium, Grapefruit, Juniper or Rosemary in the bath, and also doing skin-brushing, frequently stroking your limbs up from the extremities towards the heart, are good methods of self-help.

HERBALISM

Probably the most valuable herb for disturbances of the second half of the menstrual cycle is Chaste Tree (*Vitex agnus castus*). The berries are used, and they help to normalize

---

COMMON PMS SYMPTOMS
Symptoms include mood changes, with irritability and/or weepiness, headaches and sometimes migraines, fluid retention, tender breasts, and deep aching in the low abdomen or thighs before and at the start of the period. This half of the cycle can also be when creativity and energy, including sexual energy, can be higher so do not automatically assume that the pre-period phase has to be awful.

---

hormone function, particularly in lifting progesterone levels – lowered progesterone is most often the trigger for the symptoms. They can be

---

COUCH GRASS
(*Agropyron repens*)

obtained in tablet form. In very large amounts Chaste Tree can give an irritating sensation under the skin; if this occurs simply stop taking it.

Herbs which have diuretic effects may be useful in giving some relief; try infusions (see page 12) of either Cleavers (*Galium aparine*) or Couch Grass (*Agropyron repens*) – yes, this scourge of gardeners does have important medicinal properties! Two other helpful herbs are Chamomile (*Chamomilla recutita*), both as a diuretic and gentle relaxant, and Lemon Balm (*Melissa officinalis*) which eases the emotional

---

SKIN BRUSHING

1 To improve lymph drainage in the legs and thighs, try daily skin brushing. Lightly and briskly brush the upper legs in an upwards direction a few times, from the knees to the thighs.

2 Then brush the lower legs upwards a few times. Repeat steps 1 and 2, always starting with the upper leg and always brushing upwards towards the heart.

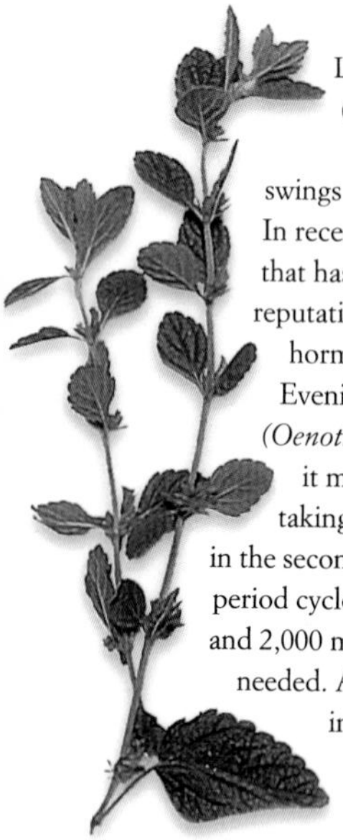

LEMON BALM
(*Melissa officinalis*)

swings that may happen. In recent times one herb that has gained a high reputation for balancing hormonal swings is Evening Primrose (*Oenothera biennis*), and it may be worth taking capsules of this in the second half of the period cycle, between 1,000 and 2,000 mg are usually needed. Any improvement in symptoms may take 3-6 months to appear.

HOMEOPATHY

Some possible remedies are:

CALC CARB: for overweight people who feel the cold easily if only during this phase, and have clammy hands and feet; may also experience tension and low abdominal pains.

CALC PHOS: for cold but drier extremities, pains and cramping, with pre-menstrual bloating.

Women for whom either of the above remedies are suited will probably get relief from pre-menstrual discomfort by taking a warm bath or using a hot-water bottle.

LYCOPODIUM: this may be appropriate when there is a good deal of pre-period irritability and tension, which quickly ease when the period starts. Abdominal

STRESS AND PMS

It can be easy to label all physical and emotional upsets as PMS (men tend to this very often), and overlook other causes of problems. Try to keep a check on whether symptoms definitely occur in monthly cycles. A good way of doing this is to keep a diary to keep a record of mood swings and general discomfort. Tension and irritability can be due to over-stress, or genuine relationship problems, which need to be sorted out. Trying to relax can also help if in a stressful situation (see also Stress, pages 28-9).

pain associated with this tension is the major physical symptom.

NATUROPATHY

Both diet and exercise can help tremendously in minimizing pre-menstrual problems. Cut down on alcohol and coffee during this part of the cycle at least, as they both affect fluid balance, and drink plenty of water to encourage kidney

EVENING PRIMROSE
(*Oenothera biennis*)

function. There has been a lot of evidence that Vitamin B6 can reduce symptoms; this is probably best taken as a supplement (up to 50 mg) as part of a whole Vitamin B complex, maybe with the addition of magnesium (200 mg). Evening Primrose oil has already been discussed earlier; for both this and Vitamin B6 it may be easier to take half the suggested doses throughout the whole of the month.

Regular exercise such as walking, cycling, swimming and running can help reduce the pelvic congestion that may accompany PMS; similarly, splashing hot and cold water around the lower abdomen regularly will improve circulation (see also Menstrual Problems, pages 68-9).

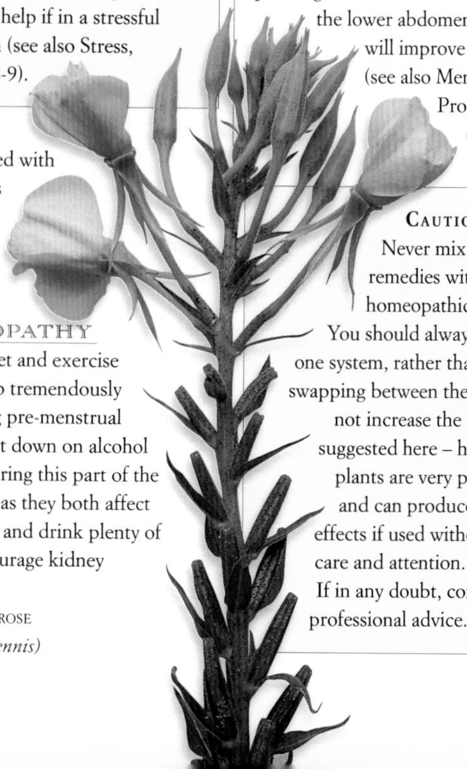

CAUTION

Never mix herbal remedies with homeopathic ones. You should always keep to one system, rather than swapping between the two. Do not increase the dosages suggested here – herbs and plants are very powerful and can produce adverse effects if used without due care and attention.

If in any doubt, consult professional advice.

PROSTATE PROBLEMS

The prostate gland is situated at the base of the bladder, and produces part of the seminal fluid. It surrounds the urethra, but normally causes no problems for urine flow. It is roughly the size of a walnut, but a common condition as men get older is a benign enlargement. This leads the prostate to compress the urethra, and perhaps even the bladder, and urine flow becomes slower to start and/or stop, with some dribbling.

AROMATHERAPY

To be used only as an adjunct to seeking professional treatment. Where there is benign prostate enlargement causing some difficulty in passing urine, placing a hot compress (see page 15) using a few drops of oils of Chamomile, Juniper or Pine over the low abdomen can quickly ease the pressure and get the urine to flow better. If the prostate is inflamed, oil of Chamomile should be included due to its anti-inflammatory effect.

HERBALISM

For an enlarged prostate, an infusion (see page 12) of one or both of the following remedies can help a good deal:
HORSETAIL *(Equisetum arvense)*: a strong

SCOTS PINE *(Pinus sylvestris)*

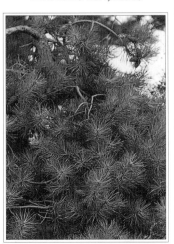

INFLAMMATION OF THE PROSTATE

Another problem can be prostatitis, or inflammation of the prostate, possibly due to a low-grade infection, and this can produce frequent, uncomfortable urination and tenderness of the gland itself. More rarely, although important to bear in mind in older men, prostate cancer can occur. This is, of course, outside the scope of self-treatment; it may be symptomless for some time, until the swollen gland restricts urine flow.

diuretic, increasing urine flow and helping the bladder to empty itself completely – failure to do so can lead to cystitis. It is also astringent and anti-inflammatory, toning the swollen membranes.
WHITE DEADNETTLE *(Lamium album)*: another astringent remedy, which seems to have a regulatory effect on blood flow through the pelvic area, and so can reduce excess swelling of the prostate.

These two herbs combined can soothe the membranes and improve urine flow.

Benign prostate enlargement is often associated with lowered testosterone levels, and Saw Palmetto *(Serenoa serrulata)* is a very useful herb in this context. The berries not only have a diuretic and urinary antiseptic effect, but they also have a hormonal action to address the underlying problem. A

decoction (see page 12) is strongest, but the berries could be taken with one or both the other suggested herbs in infusion form.

HOMEOPATHY

Some possible remedies are:
APIS MEL: when there is inflammation, probably with some enlargement, so that there is a frequent desire to pass water, but with only small amounts of stinging, burning urine.
BELLADONNA: when urination is also painful and difficult; the pressure causes some involuntary dribbling of urine when standing or moving around.
PULSATILLA: for frequent, urgent need to pass water, slight dribbling, or incontinence with any movement such as coughing, laughing or sneezing.

NATUROPATHY

Stick to a varied wholefood diet, with plenty of fluids during the day to keep urine moving through the bladder, but reduce coffee, tea or alcohol which can all irritate. Zinc is of special benefit to the prostate. Pumpkin seeds are a good food source and a supplement (up to 20 mg) may be needed daily for a while if symptoms of enlarged prostate develop.

Hydrotherapy treatment is a valuable aid; use alternating hot and cold water for the low abdomen (3 minutes hot and maximum 1 minute cold), either using a shower or splashes in the bath. The ideal method is using Sitz baths, as in hydrotherapy spa clinics.

THRUSH

Thrush is the common name for a fungal infection of the mucous membranes by the yeast *Candida albicans*. It can affect the mouth, and this is sometimes seen in tiny babies, or around the anus or on the penis, but most commonly it is a vaginal infection. A number of things can trigger off an attack of thrush; one of the major causes is often a course of antibiotics, which seriously destroy our helpful, defensive bacteria.

AROMATHERAPY

One of the most significant natural anti-fungal agents is essential oil of Tea Tree. This is available in pessary (insertable) form in some countries, but the oil can be used in the bath or in more concentrated form in a hand-basin of water; use 6 drops in warm water and bathe the vaginal area with it. Although Tea Tree oil is much more soothing than most anti-fungal drugs, do use it well diluted at first in case of any irritation. Other useful oils to use in this way are Lavender and Myrrh, and they could be blended with Tea Tree to help speed up healing.

HERBALISM

Herbalists will probably give much of the advice discussed under Naturopathy below, and are equally likely to recommend the above oils for local use; other herbs that have healing, soothing and anti-fungal effects include Marigold (*Calendula officinalis*) and Cone Flower (*Echinacea angustifolia* or *E. purpurea*). These are best used in tincture form (see page 14); dilute at the rate of 5 ml (1 tsp) to 600 ml

LAVENDER (*Lavandula angustifolia*)

OTHER POSSIBLE CAUSES OF THRUSH

Quite often a vicious circle can be set up by an infection: cystitis – treated by antibiotics – leading to thrush. Other factors can be the contraceptive pill, frequent digestive infections, a diet high in sugars, or generally being over-stressed and run-down. Conventional treatment involves the use of anti-fungal creams, or pessaries; both of these treatments may be irritating to the membranes, and self-help measures can often be the best route to avoid repetition of the infection.

(1 pt/2½ cups) of warm water, and use as a local wash. For oral thrush in babies apply a little with a cotton bud (swab), and in adults use 5 ml (1 tsp) of the tincture in a little water as a mouthwash. A powerful internal anti-fungal remedy is garlic, and if thrush recurs frequently, taking either fresh garlic or garlic capsules daily can help to combat general yeast infection. It can also be used locally, although it may irritate the vaginal

membranes if they are very inflamed – peel a clove of garlic, dip it in olive oil (you may want to tie a piece of cotton thread around it, so you don't lose it inside!), insert in the vagina and leave overnight.

HOMEOPATHY

Treatment will focus on internal remedies, backed up by local self-help measures (see next page). Practitioners may even prescribe homeopathic doses of *Candida* itself, but some other possible remedies are:
MERC SOL: for reddish patches, especially if oral thrush when there may be blisters on the mucous membranes, with thick, slimy discharge and some mould-like odour.

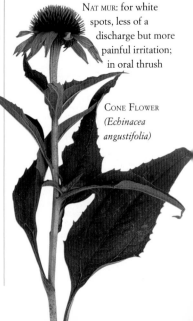

NAT MUR: for white spots, less of a discharge but more painful irritation; in oral thrush

CONE FLOWER (*Echinacea angustifolia*)

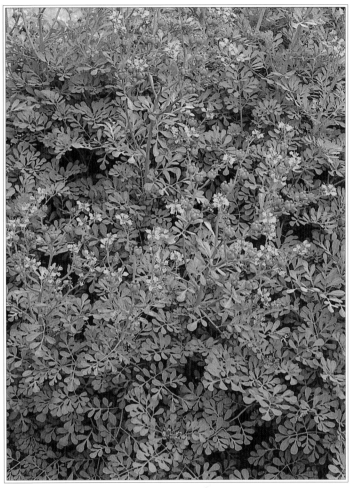

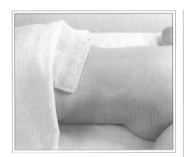

Compresses can stimulate circulation and reduce inflammation.

BRYONIA: for stiffness and swelling, for instance of the hands and arms; if the joints feel uncomfortable and "crack" with movement, this remedy may well be very useful too.

RHUS TOX: for the typical stiffness pattern of rheumatic disorders, aggravated after resting and improving after some movements. The remedy for lumbago, with low back pains on rising or after long periods of sitting.

RUTA GRAV: for pains felt in the tendons and muscles, and joints such as wrists, knees and ankles. May also be helpful in relieving sciatic pains (see page 25).

ARNICA *(Arnica montana)*

RUE *(Ruta graveolens)*

NATUROPATHY

Often a good soak in a hot bath (perhaps with a handful of Epsom salts) eases the stiffness and aching of muscular rheumatism, but too frequent a use of hot applications may produce too much congestion, so try alternating hot/cold compresses, if you can, in order to stimulate blood flow. A brisk rub with a thick, coarse towel will certainly aid this process. It is important to keep active as far as possible, so exercise is to be encouraged within individual limits of ability. Diet should be aimed at reducing acid waste matter, with plenty of vegetables and fresh fruit (with the probable exception of oranges) and very little refined carbohydrates or sugary foods. A supplement may be useful: take a multi-vitamin and mineral tablet once a day, or else initially just take a Vitamin B supplement. In winter, especially in cooler climates, taking a fish oil supplement such as cod liver oil capsules may ease stiffness.

THE SKIN

The natural approach to skin problems starts by taking the view that most disorders of the skin reflect inner imbalance, and that the whole person needs to be treated for truly effective results. This is especially so in conditions such as eczema or psoriasis, which can be highly complex disorders requiring professional treatment on an individual basis. Chronic or persistent problems should be referred to a practitioner. Given the potential negative effects of orthodox treatments such as steroid cream for eczema, there is much to be gained by looking at natural therapies.

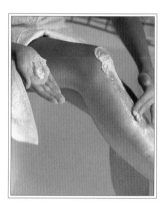

The traditional treatment of many skin problems involves considerable attention being paid to the cleansing of the whole body. Both Western and Eastern (for example, Chinese or Indian) systems of herbal medicine have developed successful strategies for treating the skin. The role of other factors such as hormone balance, stress and lowered vitality also needs to be considered; for self-help other sections of this book may therefore be very useful.

As with all the conditions discussed in this book, do not overdo any of the self-help treatments suggested; if any skin problems get worse or continue for more than a short time, then stop the treatment and/or get professional help. Do not mix therapies; this is particularly true of homeopathy since the pattern of individual symptoms will be affected by other treatments, making the choice of homeopathic remedy more difficult. Small is beautiful in all the therapies – if a dose of something is helpful, do not think that doubling the dose will have double the benefit; quite often it is the opposite!

ABOVE: Herbal creams and ointments can bring relief to problem skin sufferers.

BOILS

A boil is an acute inflamed and infected area on the skin, often in a blocked hair follicle. If a number of boils occur together, they may produce a large inflamed lump with several pus-filled "heads", and are termed a carbuncle (the medical term for a boil is a furuncle; if they are recurring, you are suffering from furunculosis). A stye is effectively a boil occurring in the base of an eyelash.

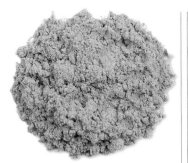

SLIPPERY ELM *(Ulmus fulva)*

AROMATHERAPY

In order to keep the tissues surrounding the boil clean and free from bacterial infection, it is very useful to wash the area 2 to 4 times a day with a 2 per cent dilution of essential oil of Lavender in cooled, boiled water, using sterile cotton wool (cotton pad) if possible. For drawing out the boil, a hot compress (see page 15) with oils such as Bergamot, Chamomile, Lavender or Tea Tree will be useful. These are variously antiseptic, anti-inflammatory and speed up healing; they may additionally be used in the bath as more general detoxifying remedies. The oil of choice would probably be Lavender; this is the most versatile oil to have for home use.

CAUSES OF BOILS

Boils tend to occur when people are run-down, either by stress or through poor diet and hygiene, but can be more frequent in some other illnesses, such as diabetes when the higher blood sugar levels provide food for bacteria (see also treatment suggestions for Abscess and Acne, pages 91 and 92-3). Generally, treatments are geared initially towards bringing the boil to a head and allowing it to burst and discharge the pus. It is important that all external applications are as clean as possible – for example, use sterile dressings for applying any poultices. In the medium to longer term, the natural therapies are ideally suited to cleansing the system as a whole, building up immunity to further outbreaks and restoring health and vitality.

Deeper causes of lowered vitality, such as prolonged stress, will need attention too, and oils may be used in the bath or in massage to help restore normal functioning. For additional help with stress, see pages 28-9.

BURDOCK *(Arctium lappa)*

LAVENDER *(Lavandula angustifolia)*

HERBALISM

Treatment from a herbal practitioner will focus internally as well as on any local applications, and this is also a good approach for self-help – if boils recur or resist home treatments, seek professional advice. Many herbs are soothing and anti-inflammatory when used as a poultice (see page 15); two excellent ones are Slippery Elm *(Ulmus fulva)* and Marshmallow *(Althea officinalis)*.

Slippery Elm has been called the "herbalists' knife" for its ability to bring a boil to bursting point; simply thicken the powder with a little boiling water and apply as a paste, as hot as you can bear. Powdered Marshmallow root can also be used, or else the fresh leaves can be softened with boiling water and applied as a hot poultice. When the boil has burst, wash the area with cooled Lavender *(Lavandula vera)* tea or else keep using Slippery Elm as a cool poultice to speed up healing. If no other herbs are available, use fresh Garlic *(Allium sativum)* on the inflamed area, gently rubbing a cut clove over the skin.

Internally, Garlic may also be helpful, as a powerful antibiotic and immune-booster. Blood-cleansing herbal remedies include Burdock *(Arctium lappa)*, Yellow Dock *(Rumex crispus)* and/or Dandelion Root *(Taraxacum officinale)*, all most effectively taken as decoctions (see page 12), and Cleavers *(Galium aparine)* or Red Clover *(Trifolium pratense)* made as infusions (see page 12). It may be valuable to take Cone Flower *(Echinacea angustifolia* or *E. purpurea)* tablets or drops for a couple of weeks afterwards to help restore natural immune function.

HOMEOPATHY

Remedies to choose from are:
BELLADONNA: for very reddened skin probably in the earlier stages of developing a boil when it is throbbing and feels burningly hot to the touch.
HEPAR SULPH: for a hot, pus-filled boil which is coming to a head; this remedy will help it to mature and burst.
SILICA: this remedy is appropriate when the boil, although painful, feels if anything cold to the touch. This remedy

MARSHMALLOW *(Althea officinalis)*

and the previous one, with their differing symptom patterns, can be thought of as the "homeopath's knife", helping the boil to discharge.

NATUROPATHY

The diet definitely needs to be overhauled in the short term at least, to clear waste matter out of the system and provide essential nutrients for the immune defences to do their job properly and to aid tissue healing. If possible, try to have a strict diet for a week, cutting out all sugar, refined carbohydrates, tea,

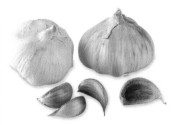

GARLIC *(Allium sativum)*

coffee, alcohol, cheese and fried foods; eat plenty of fresh vegetables, raw or cooked fresh fruit, whole grains and a little lean protein.

Fluids should mostly be water, especially spring water, or else fruit juices (diluted in hot weather) or herbal teas. Alcohol should be avoided if at all possible.

There may be a case for taking extra nutrients in the form of a supplement: if the diet has been poor for a while, take a high quality multi-vitamin and mineral supplement, or else try taking zinc, up to 25 mg daily for a week and then 15 mg daily for another month.

Locally, bathing the boil in hot water may bring it to a head, or use a hot poultice (see page 15) made from the outer leaves of a cabbage, roughly chopped.

If boils recur, or continue, then seek professional help.

Fresh green salad leaves can greatly assist in clearing out the system.

IMPORTANT NOTICE

All the treatments suggested in this book are deemed safe and have been used by professional practitioners for many years. However, any treatment could cause an adverse reaction in an individual, and if this happens to you, stop the treatment immediately and seek professional advice. Do not try self-diagnosis or self-help treatment on any

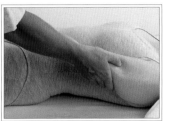

prolonged or serious problem without seeking medical advice or talking to a professional practitioner. Do not begin a course of self-help treatment when undergoing a prescribed course of medical treatment without seeking medical advice first.

Detailed below are some important reminders regarding the application of aromatherapy, herbalism and homeopathy treatments at home.

AROMATHERAPY

Essential oils should never be taken internally except under strict professional supervision. Do not increase the dosages suggested in this book. Essential oils are very powerful and doubling the number of drops is much more likely to do you harm than good.

Many essential oils should not be taken during pregnancy. Only use the doses recommended in the section on Reproduction and avoid the list of essential oils listed on page 64. All the dosages recommended in this book assume a dropper that gives 20 drops to 1 ml.

HERBALISM

As with aromatherapy oils, it is important to limit yourself to the dosages suggested herein – exceeding the dosages may cause more harm than good.

If pregnant, or likely to become pregnant, only use the herbs recommended in the section on Reproduction, and seek professional advice if in any doubt. Specific herbs to be aware of are:

SAGE: Avoid therapeutic doses if pregnant, or likely to become so. Sage should also be avoided by epileptics as sage contains thujone, which may trigger fits.

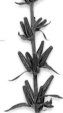

COLTSFOOT: Although there is no medical evidence of Coltsfoot causing liver damage in humans, some rats who have been exposed to large amounts of the herb have had liver damage. It should be taken internally only for a short period of time and preferably under professional guidance.

RESTRICTED HERBS IN AUSTRALIA AND NEW ZEALAND: The sale, supply and use of Borage, Coltsfoot and Comfrey is restricted in New Zealand and in some states of Australia.

HOMEOPATHY

Do not mix herbal or aromatherapy remedies with homeopathy – you will only confuse the treatment. It is also important to take the correct dosage as stipulated in this book. Potencies over 30c should always be checked by a professional before taking.

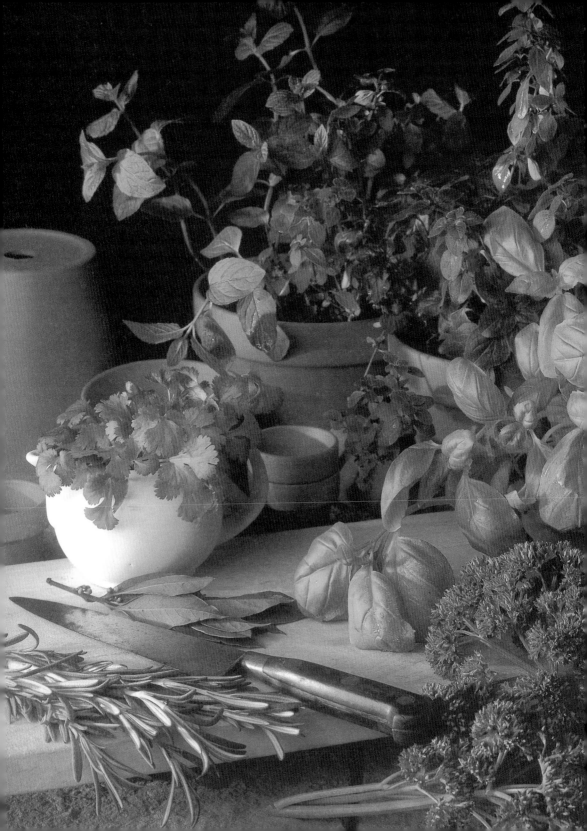

NATURAL THERAPIES

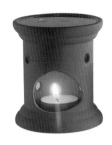

In a world of ever-increasing technology and machine-controlled medical interventions, people are beginning to feel the need for a human, individual touch; for a more natural approach to health that seeks to enhance life rather than dissect illness into more and more obscure diseases. Fortunately, there are a number of natural therapies which have just such a positive, holistic approach, and have also stood the test of time, to emerge as the most rational way to sustain our health into the twenty-first century. In the second section of this book the natural therapies are explored in five broad categories: Health from Plants covers herbal medicine, aromatherapy, the Bach Flower Remedies and Homeopathy; Naturopathy explores diet and exercise; Stress Management explains self-hypnotism and meditation as well as pyschotherapy, autogenics and healing; Bodywork offers detailed step-by-step routines in massage and reflexology, and the final category, Eastern approaches, covers shiatsu, makko ho, yoga and moxibustion with exercises that will introduce you to the benefits and theories of each discipline.

We have become accustomed to thinking of medicine as a crisis treatment for when we are sick, but one of the strengths of these therapies is their value in countering the effects of stress and helping to actually prevent illness. By reducing the impact of worries and stresses, many natural systems of treatment work to restore our vital energy and inner harmony. Eastern cultures have retained a strong tradition of therapies aimed at balancing energy, and in recent years these have gained increasing attention in the West. Our own traditional forms of treatment, such as herbalism and massage, have also undergone a resurgence in popularity, and there are the beginnings of major research projects to confirm their value. Natural therapies not only have a long history, they have a bright future.

HEALTH FROM PLANTS

The most basic and the most pervasive source of medicines throughout the world ever since time began has been the plant kingdom. From our earliest origins we can trace the use of plants for health; even today most people rely on herbal medicines for most of their primary health care.

In ancient cultures, diet and medicine were inextricably linked – let your food be your medicine, and your medicine be your food – and the importance of diet to health is discussed in another section, but plants provide an additional healthy element to our food. Herbs not only enhance the flavour of what we eat, but often contain useful trace elements and also help with the digestion of many foods. Herbal teas are low-caffeine drinks that carry many health benefits too.

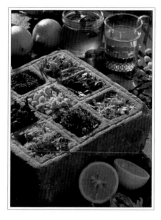

Professional herbal medicine may use plants with quite profound effects on our systems, while other therapies such as homoeopathy utilize the energetic qualities of plants, among other substances. In aromatherapy, the essential oils of plants are used to affect our emotional states, as well as for quite powerful anti-infective properties. As well as these therapies, requiring treatment from qualified practitioners, the plant world also offers many home remedies, and equally importantly plants can be used in many ways to maintain good health. This section shows some of these ways, and when to seek help.

ABOVE: A selection of herbs and dried flowers used in teas and tisanes.

OPPOSITE: A garden overflowing with plants used for centuries for their health-giving and medicinal qualities.

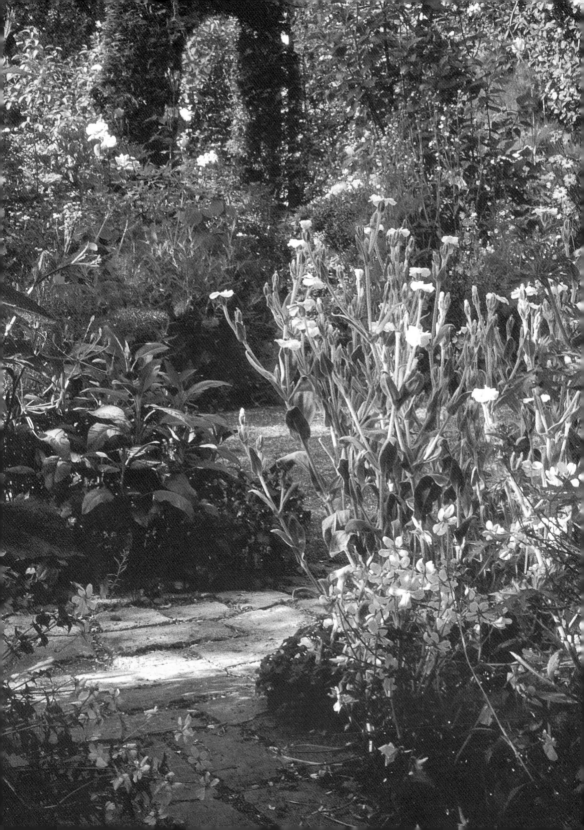

HERBAL MEDICINE

HISTORY AND ORIGINS

The history of herbal medicine is really the history of humankind, for every culture throughout time has relied upon herbs for its medicines. Some cultures – for instance, in India and China – have maintained a strong, unbroken tradition of herbalism for several centuries, while in Europe and North America its popularity has soared and plunged periodically as Western medicine achieved greater prominence. Today, however, interest in herbal medicine has increased once more, with an appreciation of its safer, holistic approach.

Probably the first system of herbal medicine, apart from the almost instinctive use of plants for healing that existed from the dawn of history and is still practised by remote tribes, was developed in India well over 4,000 years ago.

From India, the use of plants probably travelled with

RIGHT: Ma-Kou (a Chinese goddess) carrying her medicinal herbs.

migrating people into China; traditional Chinese medicine has developed a strong philosophical viewpoint on health and disease, with treatments ranging from herbal medicines to acupuncture, moxibustion and massage techniques.

Knowledge also travelled westwards, into the Middle East, and one of the significant influences on present-day European herbalism was the ancient Egyptian tradition. Papyri dating back some 3,500 years indicate that the Egyptians used several hundred plants for food and medicine. These two uses were inextricably linked for centuries, as one Greek writer put it: "Let your food be your medicine, and your medicine be your food."

As the ancient Greeks expanded their empire, so their knowledge and use of herbs was spread throughout the realm, and other plants were added to their *materia medica*. When the Romans superseded the Greeks, their army doctors carried herbs and herbal medicine all over the known world. A large number of Mediterranean herbs were thus spread through Europe and into Britain. During these two great civilizations, several major works were written on natural history and medicine which were to be fundamental to medical thought for centuries.

After the decline of the Roman Empire, much of its literature went eastwards to Byzantium and the Arabic cultures. Traditional medicine here has retained a good deal of this ancient philosophy, and some of it came back to Europe with the Moorish invasions.

After the printing press was invented, all the old Greek

BELOW: Although drying herbs alters their colour and flavour some, such as rosemary and thyme, keep many of their properties.

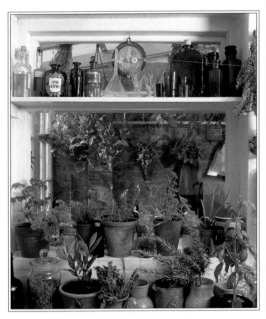

RIGHT: A traditional monastic layout is recreated in this twentieth-century garden, well stocked with a wide variety of herbs. Medieval monks kept physic gardens, growing herbs to make medicines for themselves and the local people, while the villagers would generally use simple plant treatments for all manner of ailments.

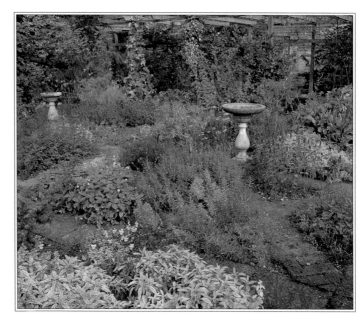

and Roman texts could be reproduced for a much wider readership. This coincided with the rapid expansion of towns and cities, and for the next three hundred years or so, knowledge and interest in herbs, in all areas of life, was greatly increased. By the sixteenth century, books about herbs were being published in the contemporary languages rather than Latin, and herbalism was an integral part of life. Books by authors such as Matthiolus, Turner, Gerard and Culpeper became bestsellers with practical advice on the uses of herbs; indeed Culpeper has never been out of print to this day, for over three hundred years.

Meanwhile, herbal medicines had been taken over by the settlers to America and used much as in Europe. It is possible to trace the spread of herbs along the eastern seaboard of the United States of America from early plantings by these settlers. Some of the more inquisitive migrants tried to learn from the Native Americans, since they were, before the importation of different diseases by the colonists, a healthy race.

The Native American system of health relied upon the use of herbs, simple yet nourishing food, fresh air and exercise. They also successfully used heat and water applications such as sweat lodges – teepees heated by a fire – with their physical and spiritual benefits.

The last ten to twenty years have seen another great resurgence in interest in natural medicine, and herbalism is both highly popular and increasingly respected as a safe and effective system of general medicine.

While today's professional practitioner of herbal medicine may see a wide range of people, often suffering from serious and chronic ill-health, the emphasis is always on the individual, looking at the whole picture of a person's health and not just any specific symptoms; this holistic approach is one good reason for its renewed popularity. Herbalism is also equally concerned with prevention or maintaining good health outside times of illness, and it is this aspect which attracts many people to use herbs in their daily lives.

LEFT: Native Americans used sweat lodges – teepees with a fire inside – as part of their natural medicine treatments.

HERBS IN FOOD

A number of widely used herbs have appreciable amounts of vitamins, minerals and trace elements, and can be thought of almost as nutritional supplements. Many others have excellent digestive qualities, helping the body cope with oily, fatty or gas-producing foods. For these reasons, as well as the extra pleasure given by their flavour, one of the earliest and best uses of herbs to help maintain health is in one's food.

LEAFY HERBS

BASIL, BAY, CORIANDER LEAVES, MARJORAM, MINT, OREGANO, PARSLEY, ROSEMARY, SAGE, SORREL, THYME.

These plants are essential ingredients in many culinary traditions, for their flavour and digestive properties. Most of these leafy herbs aid digestion, stimulating the production of enzymes that help break down fatty foods and aid absorption.

Mint sauce for example, traditionally used with lamb, helps to make this fatty meat easier to digest. Rosemary is often used with similar dishes for the same reason, stimulating the liver to work more effectively. Soups and stews are made much more tasty by the use of bay, marjoram or thyme; their aroma gets the digestive juices flowing before you have started the meal.

BASIL *(Ocimum basilicum)*

Most of these herbs contain important trace elements, and

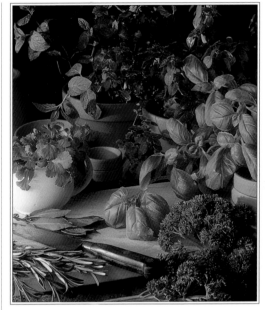

ABOVE: *Leaves such as rosemary and parsley are essential in many culinary traditions for their flavour and as aids to digestion.*

if the diet is restricted or lacking in nourishment then these nutrients can be very important in maintaining health. The herbs then become foods in themselves, and may be used in larger amounts such as in a sauce.

Parsley for instance is rich in iron and other minerals, while sorrel is a useful source of Vitamin C. Neither should be used all the time, but may add to the nutritional value of a meal. Like many other herbs, sage is a mild antiseptic and has a wide medicinal application in liver disease and respiratory tract infections. The oil is used in both the pharmaceutical and culinary industries.

CORIANDER *(Coriandrum sativum)*

The best way to benefit from herbs is to grow them yourself so that you always have a fresh supply. All the herbs mentioned above are easy to grow. You can even grow herbs inside on a sunny windowsill. Concentrate on the more common ones first and expand your collection as you go.

BELOW: *Sage, mint, rosemary and chives; herbs used in fresh and dried form for cooking and in salads.*

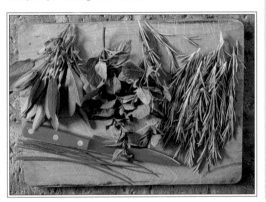

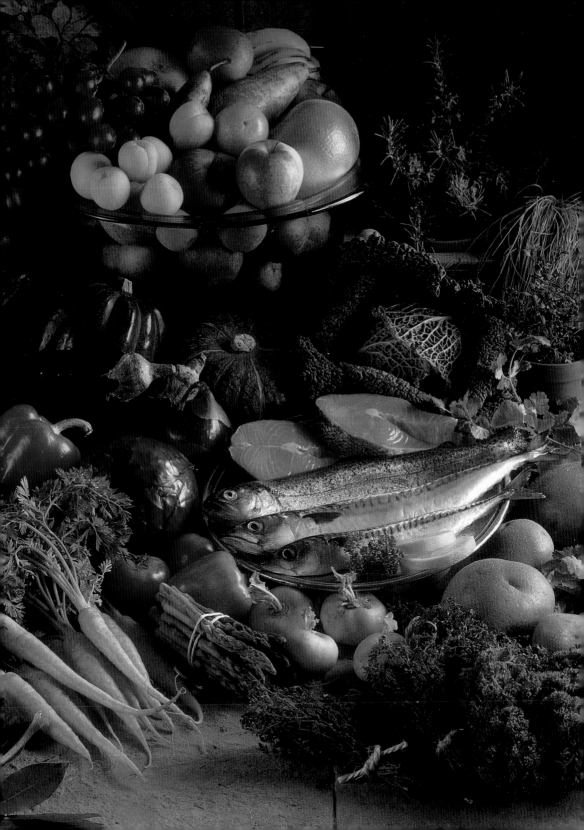

DIET AND EXERCISE

Probably the two most obvious and successful ways in which we can affect our health are through nutrition and exercise. Most of the natural therapies will include an assessment of and advice about these areas; indeed naturopathy focuses largely on them as a means of treating illness. A healthy diet and adequate exercise are essential for health, and although many books and magazines are devoted to encouraging us to work on these factors, they provide so much advice and differing theories and methods that it seems difficult to fulfil these aims.

A healthy diet involves eating foods that provide all the nourishment that our bodies need for growth, tissue repair, energy to carry out vital internal processes and to stay fit and active. In the last hundred years or so, the changes in eating habits in many countries have meant that large numbers of people have become overfed. Ironically, at the same time these dietary changes have left a lot of us undernourished, lacking in vitamins, minerals and trace elements that would help us to be in the peak of health.

Eating for health does not have to mean switching to a fussy, complicated diet, or adopting every new fad that comes

BELOW: Most people find it more stimulating to exercise in a group and there are many different classes to choose from.

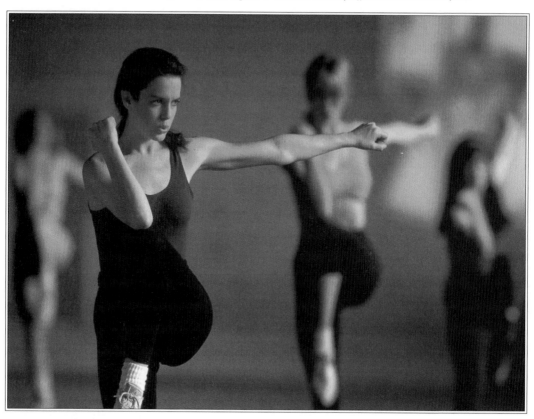

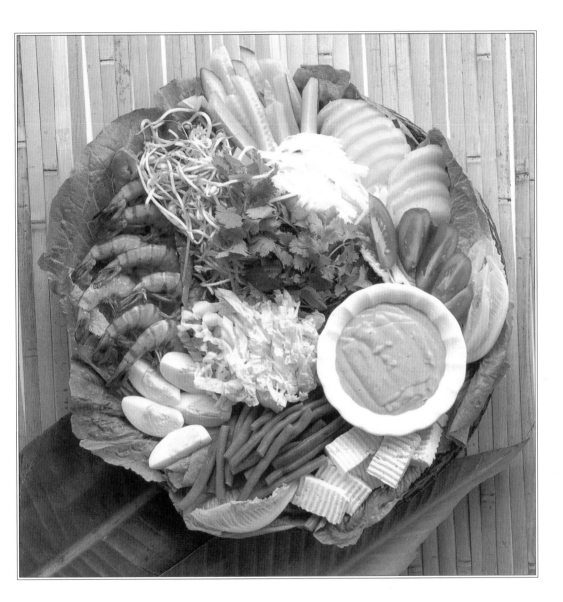

ABOVE: A healthy diet is far from boring as long as you maintain variety and imagination in your food preparation.

along. In the first place, a healthy diet should be an enjoyable one. For conventional nutritionists, food intake is broken down into various essential ingredients, such as carbohydrates, protein, fats, vitamins and minerals; however, people generally do not think in this way but eat meals or snacks which are a mixture of various elements. What is useful is to have an understanding of which foods contain which of these ingredients, and then to look at the overall balance within the diet. Balance is probably the key word in nutrition, and it is the unbalanced nature of many Western diets that lowers vitality and may lead to ill-health. With a better understanding of the elements it is easier to create a healthy diet without too much thought and analysis.

CARBOHYDRATES

Carbohydrates are our main source of energy, and need really to form the major bulk of our diet. They are broken down in the body into glucose, and used immediately for energy or else converted into glycogen for short-term storage in the liver. An excess of carbohydrates over time will be changed and stored as fat. This is a particular danger with refined carbohydrates or sugars, which do not take much processing in the body and provide large amounts of instant energy. Since they have less starchy bulk, refined carbohydrates do not make you as full, and therefore it is easier to eat too much of them, leading to fat storage and obesity.

The main sources of unrefined carbohydrates, providing dietary fibre and trace elements, are flour and grains, beans, peas and lentils, and potatoes. With grains, this is especially true when they are unprocessed, like wholegrain bread, whole oat cereals, muesli, wholewheat pasta, brown rice and so on which supply long-term energy supplies. For more immediate energy, fresh fruit, dried fruit or vegetables such as carrots or beetroot are high in fructose, or fruit sugar. This is easily broken down by the body for energy use, and since fructose metabolism does not require insulin, it can be an essential energy resource for diabetics.

There is almost complete accord among official governmental nutrition advisers and natural dietary therapists, that carbohydrates should be the chief element in our diet. In practical terms that means eating plenty of fresh

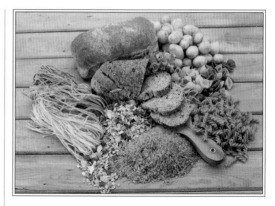

ABOVE: *Bread, rice and pasta are important for the carbohydrates which give us vital energy.*

vegetables and fruit, grains of all kinds (unless there are specific reasons for avoiding a particular grain, such as with a wheat allergy), potatoes, beans and lentils. A recent piece of advice from official organizations, for instance, has been to consume five portions of fruit or vegetables a day.

BELOW: *Eat plenty of bread, wholemeal or granary if possible.*

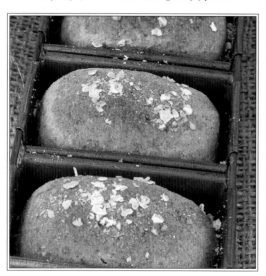

FIBRE FACTS

Fibre is important to a healthy diet. Your body cannot digest it, so, in rather basic terms, it goes in and comes out, taking other waste with it. Fibrous foods include bread, rice, cereals, vegetables, fruit, and nuts. We should aim for about 30g (just over 1oz) of fibre a day. These are some examples of good fibre sources.

GOOD SOURCES	AVERAGE PORTION	GRAMS OF FIBRE
wholemeal pasta	75g/3oz (uncooked)	9
baked beans	125g/4oz	8
frozen peas	75g/3oz	8
bran flakes	50g/2oz	7
muesli	50g/2oz	4–5
raspberries	100g/3½oz	6
blackberries	100g/3½oz	6
banana	average fruit	3.5
baked jacket potato	150g/5oz	3.5
brown rice	50g/2oz	3
cabbage	100g/3½oz	3
red kidney beans	40g/1½oz	3
wholemeal bread	1 large slice	3
high-fibre white bread	1 large slice	2
stewed prunes	6 fruit	2

PROTEINS

Proteins are the essential body-builders, helping us to create muscles, bones, tendons, hair, skin and nails. They are also vital in most of our hormone and enzyme production. The first thing to say about protein is that in most developed countries people eat too much, so the problem is not so much increasing those foods that are high in protein but getting the balance right. An excess of high protein foods in the diet will be converted into glucose for energy use or else stored as fat.

Foods rich in protein include meat, fish, poultry, eggs, milk and other dairy products, nuts and seeds, beans and lentils, and grains (bread has a little under ten per cent protein). Human protein is made from a number of simple substances called amino-acids, and these need to be present in certain amounts or combinations in the protein in our diet for us to make use of them. Animal sources do contain the right amounts of these amino-acids, but also contain relatively high levels of fat. Plant sources of proteins often need to be combined in order to give adequate levels of amino-acids; this can be something as simple as beans on toast, or a spicy bean dish with rice, and generally means having a more varied, or even a more adventurous diet.

Left: Dairy products, such as milk, butter and cheese, supply us with not only protein but also fat.

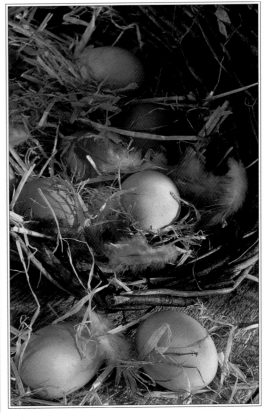

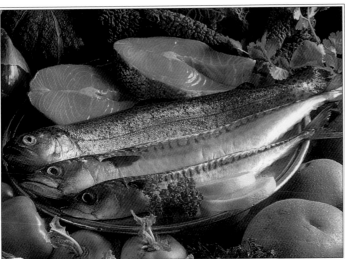

Above: Eggs are an important source of vitamins and protein but you should not eat more than two to three a week.

Left: One of the best sources of protein, fish is high in vitamins and minerals and is highly recommended by nutritionists.

Below: Eat unsalted nuts for their protein.

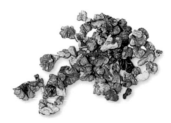

FATS

Fats are vital too, helping to form part of the cell structure and maintaining our inner organs and nerves. They also act to provide insulation and temperature regulation. It is, however, well-recognized that in the developed world much of our diet is too rich in fats, especially animal fats, and this is a major factor in heart disease, obesity and even some cancers, especially when we have such sedentary lives. Growing children, however, especially active ones, do need fats more than adults, and we should not reduce their intake so much.

Advice on fat-containing foods tends to be what to reduce rather than what to increase. Meat and dairy products can contain concentrated sources – a nice, juicy steak may have 30 per cent fat, for example. There are some differences between the effects of saturated fats (from animal products) and unsaturated fats such as are found in oily fish like salmon or plant oils like sunflower products. In general terms, move the emphasis towards the latter, using oils such as olive, sunflower, corn or safflower with salads or in cooking, but most people need to reduce all kinds of fats; they are the most concentrated sources of energy and anything over small amounts easily leads to obesity. There are plenty of reduced-fat items, particularly dairy products, which are now available and which can help in controlling fat intake.

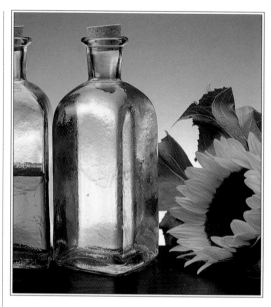

ABOVE: *Oil made from the seeds of sunflowers is an unsaturated fat which should be used instead of animal fats in cooking. Avoid frying foods, however, and grill or steam instead.*

EASY WAYS TO CUT DOWN FAT AND SATURATED FAT	
EAT LESS	INSTEAD
Butter and hard fats.	Spread butter more thinly, or replace it with a low fat spread or polyunsaturated margarine.
Fatty meats and high fat products such as pies and sausages.	Buy the leanest cuts of meat you can afford and choose low fat meats like skinless chicken or turkey. Look for reduced-fat sausages and meat products. Eat fish more often, especially oily fish.
Full-fat dairy products like cream, butter, hard margarine, milk and hard cheeses.	Choose skimmed or semi-skimmed milk and milk products and try low-fat yogurt, low-fat fromage frais and lower fat cheeses such as skimmed milk soft cheese, reduced-fat Cheddar, mozzarella or Brie.
Hard cooking fats such as lard or hard margarine.	Choose mono-unsaturated or polyunsaturated oils for cooking, such as olive, sunflower, corn or soya oil.
Rich salad dressings like mayonnaise or salad cream.	Make salad dressings with low-fat yogurt or fromage frais, or use a healthy oil such as olive oil.
Fried foods.	Grill, microwave, steam or bake when possible. Roast meats on a rack. Fill up on starchy foods like pasta, rice and couscous. Choose jacket or boiled potatoes, not chips.
Added fat in cooking.	Use heavy-based or non-stick pans so you can cook with little or no added fat.
High-fat snacks such as crisps, chocolate, cakes, pastries and biscuits.	Choose fresh or dried fruit, breadsticks or vegetable sticks. Make your own low-fat cakes and bakes.

VITAMINS AND MINERALS

Vitamins and minerals are needed for proper growth and development and body maintenance. They control the absorption of other nutrients and without them a series of complaints can develop, from headaches to sterility. There are 13 major vitamins which, apart from K and D, must be obtained from the food we eat. The fresher the food the higher its vitamin content. Food loses its vitamins through cooking, exposure to light or cold and storage, so buy small quantities of fresh food and eat it as soon as possible.

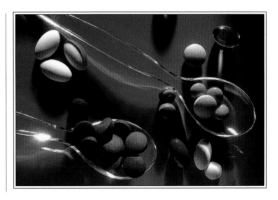

RIGHT: Supplements are an important source of vitamins but do not rely on them for all your requirements.

MINERAL AND VITAMIN VALUES

VITAMIN	SOURCES INCLUDE	BENEFITS
Vitamin A	Liver (especially fish livers), egg yolk, fortified margarine, oily fish, oranges, apricots, carrots, tomatoes, melons, dark green leafy vegetables.	Eyesight; skin; may protect against cancer.
Vitamin B1	Most foods – including wheatgerm and pulses, wholegrains, brewer's yeast, nuts, fortified breakfast cereals.	Helps break down carbohydrates; nervous system; repairs body tissues.
Vitamin B2	Brewer's yeast, liver, kidney, dairy produce, wheat bran, wheatgerm, eggs.	
Vitamin B3	Wheatgerm, wholegrain cereals, meat, fish.	Essential for tissue chemical reactions.
Vitamin B6	Avocados, liver, wholegrains, egg yolk, lean meat, bananas, fish, potatoes.	Nervous system; skin; red blood cells.
Vitamin B12	Liver, kidney, some fish (including shellfish), eggs, milk.	Healthy blood and nerves.
Vitamin C	Citrus fruits, potatoes, tomatoes, leafy greens.	Helps heal wounds, may fight colds, flu and infections; protects gums, keeps joints and ligaments in good working order.
Vitamin D	Fish liver oils, fatty fish, eggs, fortified margarine, also synthesized by ultraviolet light.	Calcium deposits in bones.
Vitamin E	Vegetable oils, some vegetables, wheatgerm.	Cell growth; antioxidant.
Vitamin K	Most vegetables – especially leafy green ones, liver.	Essential in production of some proteins.

MINERAL	SOURCES INCLUDE	ESSENTIAL FOR
Calcium	Cheese, milk, yogurt, eggs, bread, nuts, pulses, fish with soft bones such as whitebait and tinned sardines, leafy green vegetables.	Healthy bones, teeth and nails; muscle and nerve function; blood clotting; milk production in nursing mothers.
Iron	Liver, red meat, oily fish, wholegrain cereals, leafy green vegetables.	Makes haemoglobin, the pigment in red bloods cells that helps transport oxygen around the body.

HEALTHY EATING

So, what advice can be given on foods? Our needs do vary throughout life, so there is no single diet that can be suggested – thank goodness! Children and teenagers need more protein, and most other nutrients, due to their growth rates, and pregnant women have an extra need too. Hard physical work or other activity increases demand, while older and less active people may require fewer calories. What we all need is varied, healthy and enjoyable food.

Three key words are freshness, wholeness and variety. As far as possible make fresh foods the major part of your food intake – fresh fruit and vegetables, freshly cooked bread, pasta or other grains, and a little freshly prepared meat, poultry, fish or other protein-containing foods. Preparation of foods should aim to retain as much of the original goodness as possible, so grill or bake foods rather than frying them. Wholeness can be taken to indicate not just trying to use wholegrains but cutting back on processed foods as far as possible. Try to have fresh foods first, then frozen and only occasionally resort to packaged or canned food. Variety means exactly that; it is as unhealthy to eat just oranges all day as it is to eat nothing but hamburgers all day.

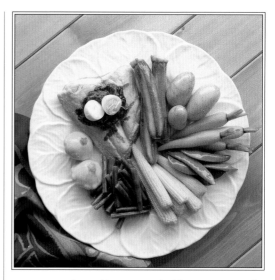

ABOVE: Steamed vegetables retain much of their vitamins as well as colour and flavour.

BELOW: Take advantage of the many kinds of fruit available around the year, and vary your intake as much as possible.

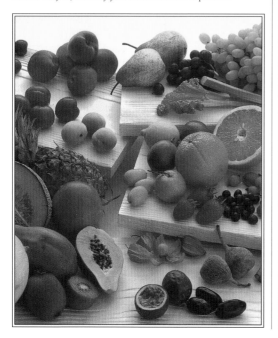

SOME IDEAS MIGHT INCLUDE:

❧ More fresh fruit and vegetables: they are high in vitamins and minerals and low in fats.

❧ Steadily increase fibre-rich foods, such as fruit, vegetables, wholegrains, beans and lentils.

❧ Eat fish, poultry and leaner cuts of meat, and avoid frying them as far as possible. Cut down on meat products such as pies, sausages and so on, which generally have high levels of fat.

❧ Eat fewer dairy products and use low-fat versions of, say, yogurt or milk.

❧ Keep pastries, cakes, biscuits and chocolates for special occasions.

❧ Drink plenty of water; many of us get dehydrated.

❧ Ease up on stimulants such as coffee and tea, and also alcohol.

❧ Try to use less salt – this also means reducing intake of processed foods, since they can often be high in salt.

❧ Enjoy food! There is a lot of pleasure to be gained from the taste and aroma of a varied diet.

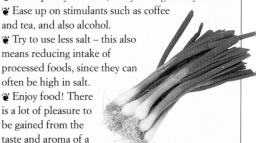

IRIDOLOGY

Iridology is the study of health and illness by diagnosing changes to the iris, or coloured part of the eye. The eyes have always been considered of some importance as indicators of internal health, or ill-health, but iridology as a distinct system dates back to the nineteenth century, to a Hungarian doctor called Ignatz von Peczely. As a boy, von Peczely had cared for an owl that had broken a wing. As the wing mended, he noticed that a thin black line which he had observed in the bird's iris gradually faded to little marks around a small dot. As an adult and a physician, von Peczely became more and more convinced through observation of his patients that similar illnesses produced similar changes and patterns of markings in their irises.

He published his findings in 1881, and they caused much interest throughout European and later American medical circles. In the 1950s in the US, Dr Bernard Jensen produced a detailed chart of the iris, locating each organ in the body to a specific part of the iris. His mapping system is quite complex, with various rings or zones relating to different systems, such as digestive, circulatory, lymphatic, muscular, skeletal and so on. Overall, the left eye shows up problems on the left side of the body, and the right eye the right side, although many disturbances seem to produce changes in both irises.

The map that Jensen and others developed divides the iris

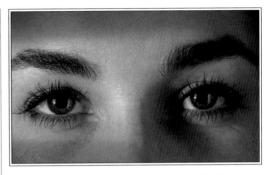

ABOVE: A healthy eye will be clear, with no signs of inflammation, soreness or discolouration.

into various sections, rather like a wheel divided by spokes. In each segment any markings within the iris are thought to be linked to different parts of the body, or else varying functions. Overlapping these divisions are the concentric rings mentioned above, which radiate from the centre of the eye outwards and are believed to show disturbances in the stomach, the glands and inner organs, the muscles and skeleton, and finally the skin and eliminative processes.

In the last 30 years or so, the knowledge of what an iris is able to show has increased, and a lot of work has been done on its complexity. There are some different schools of thought among iridologists and, in the main, although doctors find the general appearance of the eye – yellowing, dullness or unnatural brilliance, for example – an indication of ill health, conventional medicine dismisses completely the concept of specific, detailed links between parts of the body and markings in parts of the iris. Nevertheless, iridology has steadily grown in popularity among a number of therapists, who will use the technique as one of their diagnostic methods and as a non-invasive way of checking out internal functioning. An iridologist will diagnose rather than treat, and if any signs of degeneration, malignancy or disease are detected, patients are advised to see their GP.

Although many natural therapists are themselves sceptical of some of the claims of iridology, it is an area for fruitful research – our eyes are, after all, windows to the soul.

BELOW: Map of the eye showing which part relates to which part of the body.

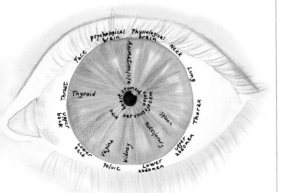

STRESS MANAGEMENT

It is probably fair to say that the greatest threat to our health today, at least in the developed countries, is having more stress than we are able to handle. The increasing pace of lifestyles, the complexity of many professions, not to mention changes and added strains in relationships due to greater mobility and thus distance from others, has placed considerable burdens on our stress-management systems.

Nearly all natural therapies place great importance on stress as a probable factor in ill-health, and yet people need a certain amount of stress in order to become motivated and develop; so what is the problem? Our internal stress-coping mechanisms originally developed to cope with potentially life-threatening situations, the so-called "fight or flight" adaptation. However, these biochemical changes are all too often brought into play by other factors nowadays, from meeting deadlines or work crises to receiving the latest bill. When the body is placed in an almost constant state of alert, the adrenal glands become tired eventually and people are depleted and panicky rather than stimulated and awake.

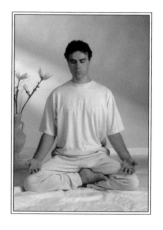

These problems have been recognized for a long time, and most natural therapies will offer some help with stress-related problems; in this section the focus is on some approaches which specialize in helping with stress-management directly.

ABOVE: Meditation is a well-known method for diffusing stress and tension.

OPPOSITE: Take time to relax and allow your body to rest during busy periods of life.

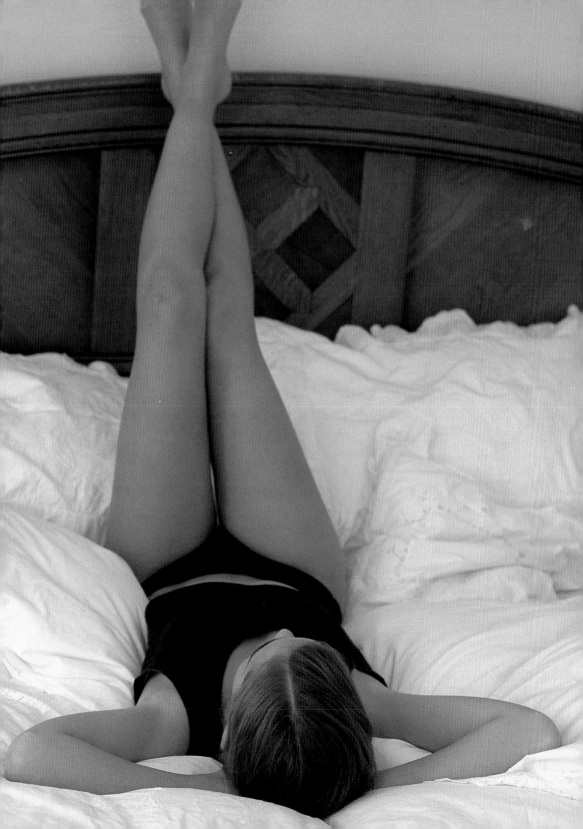

HYPNOTHERAPY

A person in hypnosis is not "asleep"; indeed they are often more aware of what is taking place than normal. Anybody (with a very few exceptions) can enter this deeply relaxed state, and indeed will, naturally.

It is believed that the state of hypnosis was used in ancient Egypt, South East Asia, and the Pacific island cultures. The hypnotic state is described in Greek and Roman writings too. The advent of Christianity appears to have marked the decline in its use, as it was then classed as witchcraft. It was, strangely enough, a Roman Catholic priest, Father Gassner, who in the late 1700s renewed public interest by using hypnotic inductions as a means of "casting out devils". Around the same time Anton Mesmer began to theorize about "animal magnetism", and the use of this phenomenon for medical purposes. He believed that Gassner was magnetizing his clients with the metal crucifix which he held. Mesmer attracted a lot of

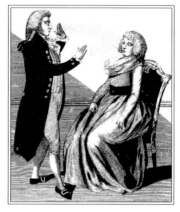

ABOVE: Mesmerism: an operator and his patient from E. Sibly's A Key to Physic and the Occult Sciences, *London.*

attention in France, and was later investigated by the French government and denounced as a fraud. It was left to James Braid to investigate further in 1841, and he is responsible for renaming mesmerism as hypnosis, from the Greek word *hypnos* meaning sleep, later trying to rename it mono-idealism, as he recognized it was not sleep but a concentration of the mind upon one channel of communication. But the words hypnosis and hypnotism had caught on, and change was impossible. Many more people after Braid developed theories about hypnosis and used it in the medical world. Perhaps the best-known exponent is a surgeon called Esdaile, who performed many serious operations painlessly using only hypnosis as an anaesthetic; some three hundred of these are carefully recorded. This method might well have continued had it not been for the discovery of chloroform and ether as chemical alternatives. It is interesting to note that hypnosis as anaesthetic is returning to popularity, especially in the US.

What then is hypnosis? It is a state of deep relaxation, a state of heightened awareness, combined with a feeling of calm lethargy. It can be best described as similar to that state between sleep and wakefulness when you are aware of your surroundings but unwilling to move. Its characteristics are a heightened susceptibility to beneficial suggestion and a much improved memory with access to "forgotten" or repressed memories stored in the unconscious mind.

In itself, the hypnotic state is very pleasant, but nothing more than that. It is very similar to the mental states achieved during meditation and yoga. It is what the therapist and client do together within this state that makes it therapy.

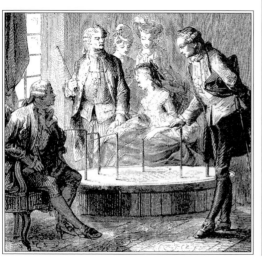

LEFT: Mesmer's tub at his consulting room in Paris which he opened soon after his treatise in 1779. The tub was a vat of dilute sulphuric acid and patients sat round it holding hands or holding on to one of the iron bars which projected from it.

SELF-HYPNOTIC INDUCTION

Self-hypnosis may not be suitable for anyone suffering from mental illness, or taking medication for a nervous condition. It is also potentially dangerous to use self-hypnosis to mask pain as this could lead to a serious illness going undetected. Ask your doctor's advice before using self-hypnosis in the above situations or if you have any doubts as to its suitability for you. It is also advisable to have one or more sessions with a properly qualified hypnotist to establish suitability and to receive instruction on how to use self-hypnosis.

Hypnosis as a natural state can be created in a number of ways, by audio, tactile or visual means. People can be shocked into hypnosis or coaxed or even bored into it. Self-hypnosis can be attained in many different ways too, but many therapists believe that by using the patterns outlined below, anyone can achieve a state of self-hypnosis. Initially, when learning these patterns, it may be useful to read them, slowly, on to a cassette tape, and then, preferably with headphones, use the tape to guide you into self-hypnosis. You may be reassured that should anything happen that requires your immediate attention, you will sit up straight away and deal with it as you would normally do: you are in control at all times. Non-intrusive music in the background can be helpful, too. Once you have learned to gain the state of hypnosis, you will be able to do so anywhere at any time that is useful to you.

STRESS MANAGEMENT

There follow three methods of self-hypnotic induction that can be highly beneficial to break a stressful day, to take five minutes to clear the mind before that important meeting, or just to unwind at the end of the day, so as to be clear thinking and able to enjoy the evening at leisure without carrying the worries of work into other areas of your life.

1 PHYSICAL RELAXATION

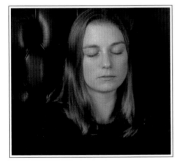 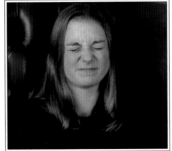 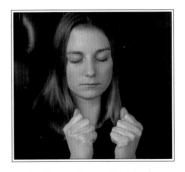

1 Settle back and relax in a chair or on a couch, or lie on your bed and just gaze upward, as if you were looking up through your eyebrows. Fix your gaze on a spot, either real or imaginary, and count down slowly from five to one. As you count down, imagine your eyelids becoming heavy, your eyes becoming tired, so that when you get to one, you can allow your eyes to close. Now begin to relax deeply. Think of the top of your head, your scalp, and concentrate on all the muscles, skin and nerve-endings there, deliberately relax them all and let go of all the tension.

2 Tense your facial muscles, scrunch them all up, around the eyes, the forehead, around the mouth, scowling and grimacing for a count of five seconds, and then release and let go, and feel that beautiful relaxation in all those muscle groups.

Thinking down through the neck and shoulder muscles and on into the tops of your arms, allow those muscles to sag down and become tension-free. Thinking over the muscles of the upper arms, tense those muscles for a count of five and let them go, let them relax down into the elbows and on to the forearms, just letting all those areas relax and let go.

3 Clench your fists, really tight, for a count of five, and release any tension, leaving the hands and arms heavy, easy and relaxed. With each breath you breathe out say to yourself, in your mind, the word "calm". Let any tension in the chest area drain away, as you think down into the stomach muscles, letting them relax too. Let all the muscles of your back relax. Thinking into your waist, your hips, and thigh muscles, let tensions drain away as you think down towards your knees … and on down into the shins and calves, allowing those muscles to relax, into the feet and toes, all muscles tension-free and feeling good.

2 THE STAIRS

Imagine a beautiful staircase stretching down in front of you made up of ten steps covered in a soft cream coloured carpet, perhaps lit with candles. Imagine you are standing on the tenth step up. Count backwards from 10 to 0, and as you count backwards, imagine each number as a step, and each step as a step down the staircase, into deeper and deeper levels of relaxation, so that by the time you get to 0, you can allow yourself to be as deeply relaxed as you can ever manage, while still aware of sounds around you.

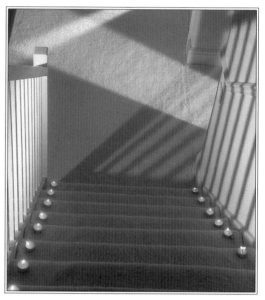

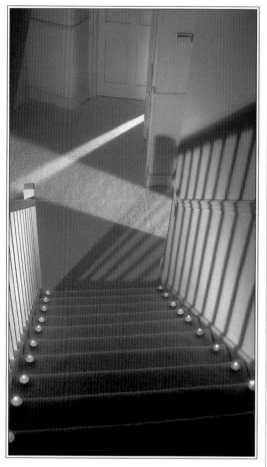

2. On step 6 you are becoming calmer ... and calmer ... even calmer still ... Halfway down the stairs and you are continuing to relax, continuing to let go and feeling good. On step 4 you are relaxing even more ... letting go ... and by step 3 – sinking deeper ... drifting further into this welcoming, relaxed state.

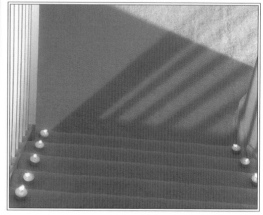

1 Imagine taking the first step down, relaxing and letting go. Take another step down, feeling beautifully at ease and at peace inside. On step 8 you are becoming more relaxed, and letting go even more ... on 7 you are drifting deeper ... and deeper ... and even deeper down still ...

3 On step 2, the last but one, you are enjoying those good feelings now, half-awake, half-asleep. By the time you reach step 1 you are nearly all the way down now, feeling beautifully relaxed. At the bottom of the staircase you are so beautifully relaxed, you can allow your mind to drift ...

3 THE HAVEN

Allow your mind to drift ... drift to a pleasant, peaceful place – a place that you know and where you can always feel able to relax completely. A safe, secure place where no one and nothing can bother you. It may be somewhere you have been on holiday, a beach or a place in the countryside. Or it may be a room you have had, one you do have or one you would like to have – an imaginary place. It's a place where you can always feel able to completely let go – a haven, a haven of tranquillity, unique and special to you.

In order to help you be in this place, notice first the lighting level. Is it bright, natural or dim, with any particular source of light – natural or manmade? Also notice the temperature level. Is it hot, warm or cool? Is there any particular source of heat? Be aware also of the colours that surround you. What are the shapes and textures and the familiar objects that make that place special?

Just be there, sitting, lying or reclining, enjoying the sounds, the smells and the atmosphere with no one wanting anything, needing anything, expecting or demanding anything from you. Now you can truly relax.

Now that you have reached that peaceful state of deep relaxation known as hypnosis, you can just relax and enjoy. You can bring yourself to full wakefulness at any time, by just slowly counting up from one to five, and allowing yourself to drift back to full physical and mental awareness, opening your eyes and getting on with the rest of your day, feeling restored and rested.

As with anything, the more you practise, the easier it will become, until you can shorten the patterns by just doing the following steps. You can achieve self-hypnosis in two to three minutes at most with these four steps.

1 Close your eyes.
2 Check that you are physically at ease.
3 Use the sound of the word "calm" with each breath you exhale.
4 Imagine yourself in your own "haven".

THE CALM TECHNIQUE

Once you have used the methods of self-hypnotic induction a few times, the mind has accepted the sound of the word "calm" as a signal for physical relaxation and mental calmness. This can then be used anywhere to control emotions and allow a return to clear thinking and just the right level of calm and relaxation for the situation. No one else will know you are doing it, but it puts you back in control. It is an ideal technique for a meeting that has become heated, and for immediately calming yourself before giving a presentation or having an interview.

BELOW: Your safe place might be a beautiful, sunlit woodland glade, with shafts of light illuminating the forest floor.

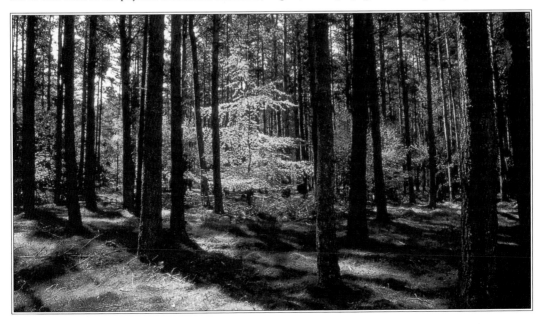

AFFIRMATIONS AND VISUALIZATION

Self-hypnosis can be usefully combined with affirmations, which have been brought into the forefront of psychotherapy in recent years. This deceptively simple device can be used by anyone and has proved remarkably effective.

It is recommended that you use this method while in self-hypnosis, having previously planned and memorized the affirmations involved. Thus you combine that ease of access to the unconscious mind and the effectiveness of repeated powerful positive phrases. You must say to yourself, out loud, a positive statement about yourself such as "I like my … (physical attribute);" "I am proud of my … (attitude or achievement);" "I love meeting people – they are fascinating;" or "I am quietly confident at meetings".

Notice the main points in these affirmations which can be used singly or together. They are in the present tense, and they are positively phrased and imply an emotional reward. You can create your own, and use them as often as you wish. The oldest and best-known affirmation is "every day in every way, I am getting better and better", written by Emile Coué at the end of the nineteenth century.

Yours is the most influential voice in your life, because you believe it. Used in this powerful combination, it can be truly effective in changing your expectations and reactions and in influencing outcomes.

In the same way that you can utilize your voice, so – and perhaps more powerfully – you can use your imagination. The imagination can stimulate emotions and can provide a direct communication with the unconscious part of the mind, and can also provide an impetus for registering new and more positive attitudes in the mind.

Visualization requires that you imagine yourself behaving, reacting and looking as you would wish to do in a given situation; for example a business meeting or a social gathering, and what that will mean for you. See your reactions, the reactions of those around you, and, most important, experience all the good feelings that will be there when this happens in reality. It is like playing a video of the event, on that screen on the inside of the forehead, the mind's eye, from the beginning of the situation through to the perfect outcome for you. Should any doubts or negative images creep into your "video", push them away and replace them with positive ones. Keep this realistic, and base it upon real information from your past.

Again the best time to do this is when relaxed mentally and physically – in self-hypnosis. Teach your mind to expect new, positive outcomes. This can be combined with affirmations and be doubly effective.

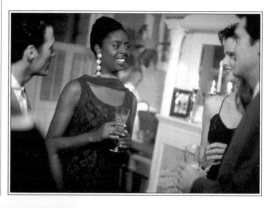

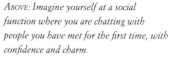

ABOVE: *Imagine yourself at a social function where you are chatting with people you have met for the first time, with confidence and charm.*

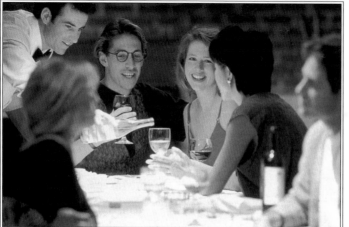

LEFT: *Imagine yourself at a social gathering, such as a dinner party, where you are relaxed, comfortable and happy. You know that others are enjoying your company just as you are enjoying theirs.*

THE SWISH TECHNIQUE

This technique is particularly useful to combat pre-interview or presentation jitters. It is a very effective method utilizing visualization and is derived from NLP (Neuro-Linguistic Programming), which is used throughout the world by therapists and patients alike. You can use this technique at any time when you feel relaxed. First thing in the morning, before getting out of bed, is a good time. Ideally, however, include this in your self-hypnosis programme and it will take just five minutes. Just work through it, with the instructions beside you, and then you will be able to do it on your own.

First, think of the event that is going to happen, an interview for example, about which you feel anxious. Focus in on that for a moment. You will probably find it much easier with your eyes closed.

Now create two pictures in your mind, filling the whole of the screen on the inside of your forehead, your mind's eye. The first picture is called "The Moment of Anxiety", and depicts the scene at the moment when you would expect to start feeling most anxious. Make the picture as detailed as you can: the room, the people, furnishings and so on – like a photograph you have taken yourself, so you are not in the picture, in full colour, detailed and brilliantly lit. When you are sure you have done that, put that picture to one side.

Next, form another picture; this one is called "The Moment of Achievement". This is a picture of you at the end of that occasion, looking really good, relaxed and happy, leaving the interview perhaps. Make this picture as detailed as you can: but most important of all – you, and the look on your face. The event has gone well and you feel really good. Make sure you have this in your mind as clearly as possible.

BELOW: The Moment of Anxiety.

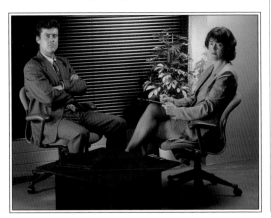

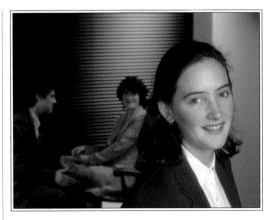

ABOVE: The Moment of Achievement.

Now see both of these pictures in the following way. The first picture, "The Moment of Anxiety", in full colour and brilliantly lit filling the whole of your mind's eye except for one of the lower corners, where, like a snapshot tucked into the frame of a larger picture, there is a small, dull black-and-white picture, "The Moment of Achievement".

When you have them clear and steady, swish them over – the small becoming large and full colour, the large becoming small and black and white. Allow yourself a few moments to really enjoy the feelings displayed on your face.

Clear your mind by opening your eyes and looking around you. Then set the pictures up again as they were before, with the Moment of Anxiety large and full colour and the Moment of Achievement as a small black and white snapshot, then swish them over. Do that exercise three more times, making five times in all.

Use the SWISH technique once a day for about a week before the situation you have in mind. You will find that very soon it is impossible for you to hold the first picture in your mind's eye without the second one automatically taking over. When this happens, you know that you have reprogrammed your mind for success rather than failure. Then repeat the exercise for two more groups of five to make absolutely sure.

It is under your control now. You can use this exercise to help yourself to gain the right attitudes so that you can be successful in many different situations.

Under no circumstances should the patterns illustrated here be used on someone else, nor should any effort be made to delve into personal history or past lives without the aid of a professional therapist. It can lead to situations that can quickly get outside of your competence.

MEDITATION

The word "meditation" means different things to different people. In the Western philosophic and religious tradition it can simply mean turning an idea or concept over in one's mind. What it has generally come to mean today is some form of clearing or emptying of the mind. A word such as "contemplation" may have been used at other times to mean the process of coming to a central point, focusing and quietening the mind. These practices are often referred to simply as "sitting".

Very often the word "meditation" is associated, in many people's minds, with all sorts of bizarre practices involving wearing long robes and sitting on the floor with your legs tied in a knot for hours on end. In short, there is a lot of mystification surrounding the idea of meditation. By describing some basic principles and aims in this chapter, and intro-

BELOW: When you are meditating make sure you are in a quiet, peaceful place with no risk of interruption or distraction.

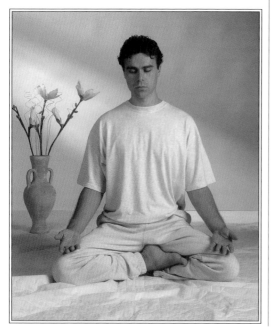

ducing some simple exercises which should benefit most people, some of that mystification should be dispelled.

There are hundreds of different schools of meditation, many associated with some form of religious practice, and many that are not. Some of these varied forms of meditation may include techniques such as complex visualizations or chanting words or sounds known as "mantras". Many of the world's great religions also make provision for retreat from the world in order to focus more closely on meditation for short or long periods. Practices of this kind have great value, but often form the basis for widely held and perhaps stereotyped ideas about what meditation involves. All of these techniques, and more, can also be practised without the necessity of being a follower of any particular religious tradition. (Incidentally, the exercises presented in this chapter are considered to be quite compatible with whatever religious belief, if any, an individual may already hold.)

Of course, you may choose to incorporate any, or all, of the above exercises into your practice, but none of them is strictly necessary in order to gain the benefits that meditation can bring to a modern, stressful lifestyle. Meditation is a truly holistic activity in that, ideally, the whole system of body, mind and spirit is involved and benefited.

BODY

The physical benefits of meditation are easily quantifiable and plenty of research documentation exists. These include relaxation, improvement of sleeping patterns, lowering high blood pressure, helping recovery from fatigue and a general beneficial effect on most stress-related disease. Posture can be helped, too, in that better posture leads to better meditation which in turn leads to better posture! The same can be said for relaxation. The mind cannot let go until the body relaxes, and vice versa.

Meditation is sometimes seen as a kind of vanishing upwards into rarefied heavenly atmospheres, rejecting all that is grossly physical. On the contrary, awareness of the body is an essential part of effective meditation. A kite can only fly if the string is firmly held on the ground. Many of the emotional stresses and upsets that people experience can be held as tensions in the body and therefore be fairly

ALEXANDER TECHNIQUE

The Alexander Technique is a method of training in posture, body movement and positioning. It was originally devised by Frederick Alexander, an Australian actor, around the turn of the twentieth century. He found that when he was giving an important Shakespearean speech on stage, his voice continually faltered. The only advice given to him was to rest his voice, which only helped until the next large role. Eventually, he set about studying exactly how he was using his body by watching himself in a mirror, and discovered that he tensed his body when performing. The effort of projecting his voice made him bring his head down, restricting his vocal cords and impairing deep breathing or voice control.

Over a period of time Alexander slowly adapted the way he held his body when acting on stage, and overcame this "startle reflex pattern" as he called it. Gradually he developed the idea that body use – how we hold ourselves, move and so forth – can affect the functioning of our internal organs and overall health. He started to teach his methods of body realignment, moving to London in 1904 and subsequently going to the US gaining widespread recognition.

The techniques he devised are based upon the principle of extending the spine, allowing it to reach its optimal length, and generally to redeploy the body's entire muscular system. Exercises are thus geared to restoring natural posture and ease of movement, with minimal muscular effort. A common phrase used to describe the ideal movement is, "the head leads, the spine follows."

Animals and young children usually move naturally, with a lengthened spine and a sense of poise. Unfortunately, we often acquire bad habits as we get older, and additional stresses can lead to imbalanced and excessive muscular effort in movement. If chronic tensions build up, the neck and back muscles contract, leading to rounded shoulders, a lowered head and an arched back, which causes further tension and so the problem gets worse and worse. Alexander teachers seek to help re-educate us to change these patterns and regain positive, easy body use.

Alexander schools have often been associated

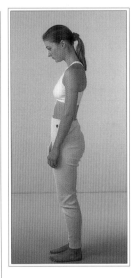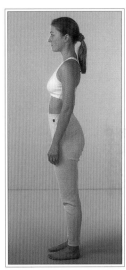

FAR LEFT AND ABOVE: The basic principle of Alexander's ideal posture is to keep your body in a straight line.

with drama or music establishments, echoing the man's background, but the techniques are suitable for all kinds of occupations. Improvements in posture can be accompanied by health benefits such as greater mental alertness, better sleep, increased resistance to stress and enhanced performance of physical tasks. The techniques are learned from a teacher, in the form of lessons rather than treatment sessions, and may initially involve simple actions such as sitting down and getting up from a chair or walking to and fro, with corrective advice on how to use the body more efficiently.

Self-help measures may be of benefit in the first instance; copying Alexander's example and looking closely at your posture in the mirror might be valuable in identifying obvious imbalances. However, since bad habits can be difficult to change, or even spot sometimes, a series of lessons from a teacher is likely to be the most helpful way to correct these.

The Alexander technique is not a cure-all, but improvements in the way we hold and use our bodies can improve many people's overall health and movement.

EASTERN APPROACHES

⊷⊶

The traditional Oriental view of health is quite different from the reductionist standpoint of modern, technological medicine in the West. In Eastern philosophy, illness is placed in the context of a holistic approach to life, and in particular the concept of an energy-based system. From the idea of a universal energy, or the highest level of spirituality, down to the lowest forms of life, much of Eastern ideology is an energetic one, with all parts of the human body interconnected and infused with a vital energy, and all life-forms similarly interdependent on an exchange of energies.

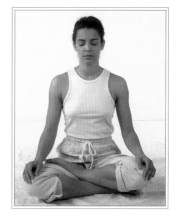

These concepts have led to the development of traditional therapeutic systems, such as acupuncture in China, shiatsu or acupressure in Japan, and yoga in India. Some of these are more suited to professional treatment of ailments, or imbalances in energy flow as they would be described, while practices such as yoga are very suitable for everyday life, in order to *prevent* illness as well as to promote self-development.

Modern medicine in many Far Eastern countries is now often an amalgam of conventional Western medicines alongside traditional approaches; they are quite happy to utilize the best of both worlds, and this is perhaps a useful pointer to the rest of us. Acute, severe illness may be treated with hi-tech medicine, but a more holistic approach can remedy most health problems.

ABOVE: Yoga is one of the most ancient ways of releasing the mind.

OPPOSITE: Acupuncture, once practised only in the East, is now available throughout the world.

LIVER AND GALL-BLADDER

The liver and gall-bladder meridians relate to the wood element and the tree's qualities of strength and flexibility when it is healthy. Try to feel these qualities in yourself, if your body feels stiff, you may be frustrated or angry.

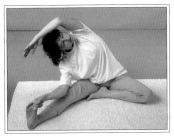

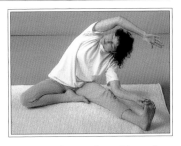

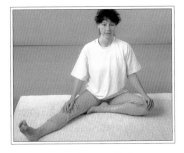

1 Sit upright with your right leg outstretched and flat on the floor; the foot is vertical to keep the knee straight. Tuck your left foot into the body. Breathe in, feeling an alive quality.

2 On the exhaled breath lean sideways over your right leg grasping your big toe if possible, keeping your leg straight, and easing your body downwards. Do not strain. Keep your chest open and your left arm close to your ear. Feel a strong stretch to the side of your body. Look upwards. Do not collapse your chest or bring your raised arm in front of your face. Breathe three times. Release on the third exhaled breath. Repeat three times.

3 Return to the upright position and then change sides with your left leg stretched out and your right foot in. Breathe in. On the exhaled breath lean sideways as before, this time to the left. Breathe three times. Repeat three times.

FINISHING EXERCISE

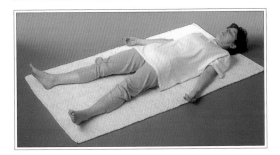

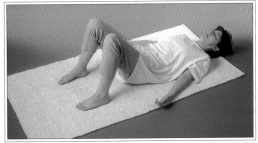

1 After you have completed the whole sequence (ideally three times plus the specific self-healing phase), lie flat on the floor with your eyes closed and just breathe gently for a few minutes, allowing everything to settle in your body.

2 You may be aware of tingling sensations as your inner energy responds to your makko ho exercise session. Another finishing position is lying flat on the floor with your knees up. Breathe into your stomach and relax.

FURTHER PRACTICE

Human nature being what it is, it is inevitable that resistances to doing these exercises will occur at some stage. You are encouraged to note your resistances and continue the exercises anyway and not to give up in the first week, before you really begin to feel the benefits of the makko ho exercises. While acknowledging the hectic pace of our lives, it can always be possible to carry out at least one sequence of exercises per day. Obviously the more time and energy you give to yourself, the greater the benefits will be. Enjoy your exploration and be well.

YOGA

The word yoga is by now well known outside India. In fact, over the last four decades it has quietly and steadily taken root in Western culture and language. Yet if you ask a number of people what yoga is, you are likely to get many different responses. These responses are sometimes contradictory. However, yoga can be summarized into the following three possibilities or approaches.

1 YOGA AS POWER

First, yoga can be explained as a means to attain a degree of power or control over the body and mind. Yoga links the body and the mind through intense physical and mental effort. For instance, through rigorous physical practices a state of concentration is developed and maintained which is used to hold power over the body and the breath. Within this approach, such control is often seen as a prerequisite to the body and mind becoming free of disturbances and distractions. This power arises out of three areas of personal development:

    i) Mastery of the body through physical postures;
    ii) Control of the breath through breathing techniques;
    iii) The ability to concentrate through mental techniques.

    This intense effort produces energy and control that is available for whatever purpose suits one's direction in life. Many people could usefully enjoy more power over certain areas of their lives. The question is whether they are prepared to put in some effort to reach this point.

    In the words of a yoga teacher from long ago: "Yoga is the means by which that which was not attained

RIGHT: Yoga is a process by which you grow in self-understanding.

earlier is now attained." This approach is known as the yoga of energy and will. As such, this aspect of yoga is an art and offers a fascinating field to explore. It appeals to many people searching for power in and over their lives. However, this approach is only a means towards a more important goal.

2 YOGA AS MEDITATION

Here the concern is more with the mystery of life rather than the mastery of life and yoga is a means for meditation with self-inquiry as the primary focus. "Who am I?" is the question that acts as a map for an inner journey into your mind. It is a quest to touch and be touched by the "soulful" quality of being that resides within a person. In this approach, yoga is a tool for a movement towards a deeper relationship with your sense of soul, by searching both into and beyond what you experience as the everyday self. It is a journey of discovery, exploring and ultimately going beyond attitudes that, for better or for worse, have shaped your life, work and relationships.

Yoga is a skill by which you seek to sustain awareness and clarity in spite of the vagaries of everyday life. The quality of this awareness engenders a freshness within which actions are less affected by the usual attitudes and habits. In other words, there is more choice over how you respond or react. In those situations where your reaction would have been automatic, there are now different possibilities.

Yoga is a process by which you grow in your understanding of yourself. From this you come to realize that you can change those aspects of yourself that are unhelpful on your journey through life. This means first recognizing the qualities that hinder your personal growth – an important, if not always comfortable, stage in the journey. Second, having reflected on how

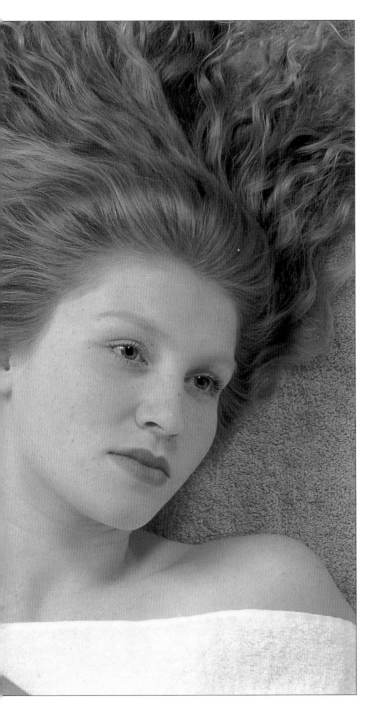

FANNING THE SHOULDERS

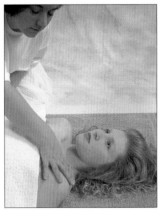

1 With fingers spread, brush with the flat of the hand across from the breastbone and out over the shoulders.

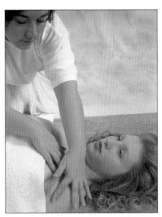

2 The second hand follows closely behind the first, so they are draining simultaneously toward the armpit.

Repeat twice before moving onto the other shoulder.

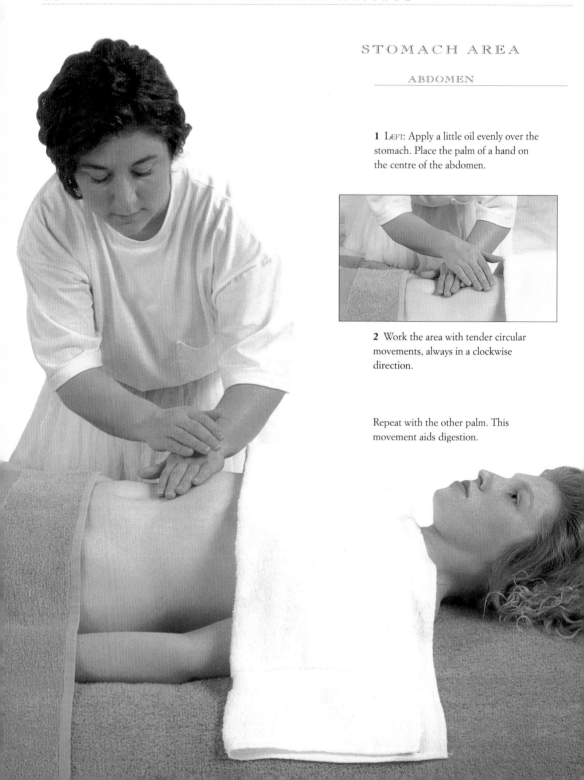

STOMACH AREA

ABDOMEN

1 LEFT: Apply a little oil evenly over the stomach. Place the palm of a hand on the centre of the abdomen.

2 Work the area with tender circular movements, always in a clockwise direction.

Repeat with the other palm. This movement aids digestion.

RIB CAGE SWEEP

This movement helps to cleanse the stomach and spleen by pushing the lymph away from these areas.

WAIST PULLS

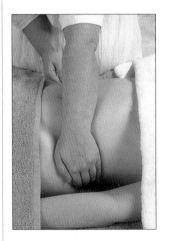 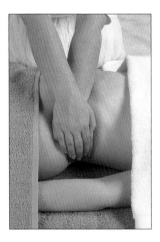

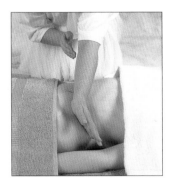

1 Starting with the outer edge of the hand placed at the centre of the rib cage, sweep away from you, following the line of the ribs with a long sweeping movement out to the waist.

1 Reach across your partner, placing a firm grip around the waist with one hand. Reinforce your grip by placing your other hand on top of the first hand.

2 Lift the waist by pulling your partner's body-weight toward you, then gently release while sliding the hands around the hipbone. This cleanses the liver and gall bladder.

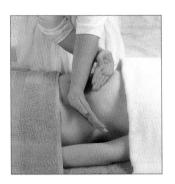 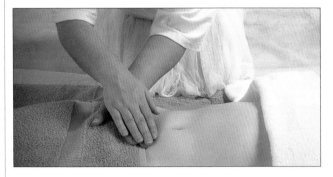

2 As the first hand finishes the movement, the other hand follows on the same side.

Repeat the movement with both hands six or seven times and then move around the body to work the other side of the rib cage.

3 Complete the movement by sliding the hands across and around the pelvis, draining toward the major glands in the groin. Be careful not to dig with the fingers as this is an extremely tender area. Keep the pressure light and even over the whole hand. This is particularly beneficial for women who suffer from menstrual problems.

Repeat five or six times before moving around to the other side of the body.

FRONT OF LEGS

EFFLEURAGE

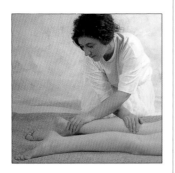

LEG STRETCH

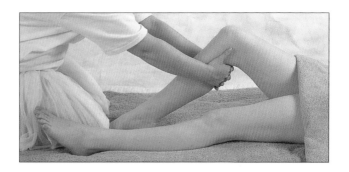

Apply oil to both legs using an *effleurage* movement working up from the ankles, as used on the back of the legs.

Repeat the *effleurage* strokes sequence several times to ensure an even distribution of oil.

Supporting the leg at the ankle and behind the knee, bend the leg up and place it in line with the shoulder.

Clasp the hands around the back of the knee. Ask your partner to inhale deeply, then pull the calf muscle toward you.

Hold for a slow count of 3. As your partner breathes out, release the pull on the calf.

Repeat the whole movement three times, then gently lay the leg down and repeat the stretch on the other leg.

ARMS AND HANDS

EFFLEURAGE

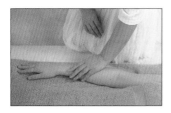

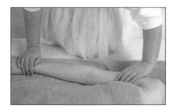

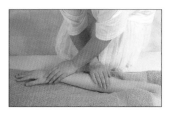

1 Seated to the side of your partner, move the arm slightly away from the body. Apply the oil by sweeping from just above the wrist, up to the shoulder and round.

2 As the first hand comes off the arm, the other hand starts at the wrist and sweeps upward to the gland sited in the elbow joint.

3 The first arm crosses the second as it reaches the elbow and again sweeps from wrist to shoulder.

Repeat six or seven times.

You can follow the *effleurage* with flushing to the inside of the arm, using the same movements performed on the leg, working from the wrist to the elbow. Before going on to the second arm, massage the hand of the first arm.

HAND MASSAGE

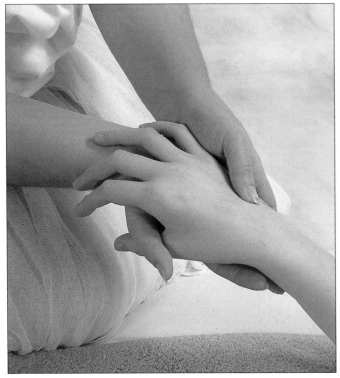

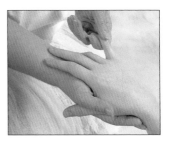

2 Pull back to the fingers, gently massaging the joints between your thumb and forefinger as you draw toward the tips. Finish with a slight pull to the finger to stretch it out.

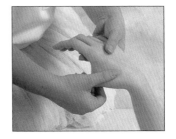

1 Resting your partner's hand palm down over your own palm, use small brushing movements with your thumbs to work upward between the joints of the fingers toward the wrist.

3 Repeat with each finger, finishing with the thumb.

Now repeat the movements on the other arm and hand.

To finish the massage, cover your partner to the neck, check he or she is warm and comfortable, and leave to rest for a minimum of 5 minutes (up to 15 minutes is preferable). Upon returning, help your partner to sit up carefully and offer a glass of water.

PREGNANCY TREATMENTS

※─═◎◎═─※

Pregnancy can be one of the most exciting and fulfilling times of a woman's life. The joy of bringing another human being into the world creates a tremendous feeling of contentment and anticipation, but it is also a time of great physical and emotional upheaval. Together with the ever-important trio of exercise, good diet and rest, essential oils can play an important role in helping a woman cope with the stresses of nine months of pregnancy, the pain of labour and post-natal recovery.

COMMON AILMENTS

Surging hormone levels and changes in your swelling body can bring a host of discomforts, many of which can be alleviated by aromatherapy treatments and other simple steps.

BACKACHE
The lower back region takes a lot of strain during pregnancy, and will benefit from a firm massage with 4 drops each of lavender and sandalwood in 30 ml (2 tbsp) base oil. 6 drops of lavender in the bath will help to soothe away the aches.

MORNING SICKNESS
Eat little and often during the day, avoiding junk food and heavy meals late at night. Choose fresh foods which are free from preservatives or chemicals. Try herbal tea infusions such as chamomile, peppermint or orange blossom, which are good for the digestion.

HEARTBURN
Avoid heavy meals and particularly rich, spicy foods. Peppermint tea infusions help, and you can rub the solar plexus with a blend of 2 drops each of lemon and peppermint essential oils in 15 ml (1 tbsp) of base oil.

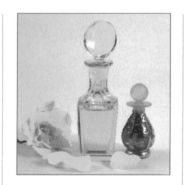

Spoil yourself with the luxurious and relaxing scent of rose for body and facial oils, to keep your spirits up during pregnancy.

SORE BREASTS
These need extra care and attention during pregnancy as they expand. Use a gentle massage oil with rose and orange, 3 drops of each in 15 ml (1 tbsp) sweet almond oil; or if breasts are swollen, make a cool compress using rose water and place over the breasts while having an afternoon rest. Sweet almond oil on its own is excellent for sore, cracked nipples during breast-feeding. Never use pure essential oils on the breasts during this period as they can easily be transferred to the baby while feeding.

CONSTIPATION
Make sure your diet contains plenty of fresh and high fibre foods and drink plenty of still water. Tension can also be a contributory factor, so try a relaxing bath with 3 drops of lavender and 4 drops of rose. Massage your abdomen and the small of the back with a blend of 4 drops of chamomile or orange in 15 ml (1 tbsp) base oil.

SLEEP PROBLEMS
In the last few months of pregnancy, because of various discomforts it is often difficult to get a good night's sleep. A relaxing bath with neroli and rose is soothing, and you can add ylang-ylang for its calming, sedative effect – a maximum of 8 drops in total. Sprinkle 2 drops of rose or lavender on the edge of the pillowcase to help induce sleep.

STRETCH MARKS
When the stretched skin returns to the body's normal shape it can leave tiny jagged scars. A daily massage around the hips and expanding tummy, using 5 drops of lavender in 15 ml (1 tbsp) jojoba, wheatgerm or evening primrose oil, will help keep skin smooth and supple. Start around the fifth month of pregnancy and continue after the birth until you return to your normal weight.

THE STIMULATING BATH

Best for the morning to get you started or to revive you before an evening out. Keep the water fairly cool and use an invigorating bath mitt to rub down and stimulate the circulation. When you have soaked, rinse yourself with water as cold as you can bear, either by splashing directly from the tap or shower, or by adding more cold water to cool down your bath.

As you get out, either slap yourself dry to make the skin tingle or rub yourself vigorously with a towel.

OILS FOR STIMULATION

Cypress • Eucalyptus • Fennel
Geranium • Juniper • Lavender
Lemon • Lemongrass • Peppermint
Pine • Rosemary • Thyme

THERAPEUTIC BATHS

OILS FOR DERMATITIS
Chamomile • Hyssop • Lavender

OILS FOR ECZEMA
Chamomile • Geranium • Hyssop
Juniper • Myrrh • Rosemary

OILS FOR PSORIASIS
Bergamot • Chamomile • Lavender

OILS FOR ARTHRITIS/RHEUMATISM
Chamomile • Eucalyptus • Juniper
Lavender • Rosemary • Thyme

SHOWERS AND COLD RINSES

Invigorating jets of water are ideal for getting the blood pumping and there is no need to forgo the benefits of aromatic oils. Skin tends to be sluggish in the cold winter months but sloughing off dead top layers can help regenerate cells and allow moisturizers to be absorbed more easily. An aromatic shower is an excellent way of aiding recovery from a certain illness, lifting the spirits, or promoting relaxation after a busy day. Showers are ideal for smoothing skin with exfoliating rubs using wet salt, a loofah or a mitt to slough off the top surface of dead skin cells. A dry friction glove or loofah is too harsh for most skins so soften first in warm water. Soft bristle brushes can also help to get the circulation going with gentle massage on problem areas like hips and thighs. To keep friction brushes and mitts fresh always rinse them well and hang up to dry.

Essential oils can be used under the shower: try a base oil mixed with invigorating essences and with a clean face-cloth or sponge, pour on the oils and rub all over the body in circular motions whilst showering. To clear the sinuses and help coughs and colds, sponge the chest with a mix of eucalyptus and peppermint oils. A cold-water shower after cleansing improves the circulation and tightens skin pores.

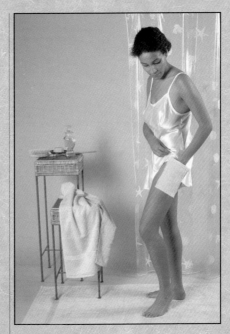

Start off your shower or bath routine by whisking off dead skin cells with a friction mitt. Moisten the palm of the mitt with warm water or softening oils such as sweet almond or evening primrose. Concentrate on outer thighs, working from the knee in upward circular movements across the buttocks.

AFTER-BATH BODY TREATMENTS

⋄⊷━◉━⊶⋄

oisturizing oils and lotions applied after the bath or shower help to nourish the skin, keeping it soft and supple. As we get older our skin dehydrates since the oil glands do not produce as much oil as in youth. Apply a body oil all over the body, starting from the feet and working right up to the neck and tips of the ears. Avoid talcum powders which clog the pores and tend to have a drying effect.

BODY-OIL FORMULA

The use of essential oils for skin care combines simple pleasure with health benefits. Essential oils sink beautifully into warm damp skin. For a lasting effect, mix the 3 chosen bath essential oils, 5 drops of each, in 30 ml (2 tbsp) base oil. If you want to make up a larger quantity of body oil, use a concentration of 3 per cent essential oil in base oil.

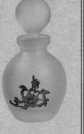

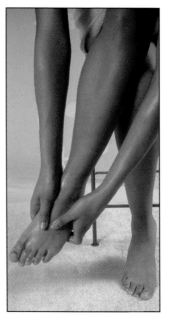

ABOVE: Condition hands and nails with a simple finger-pulling exercise. Spread and stretch the fingers straight out; massage each finger with oils, working from the tip of the nails to the cuticles and up to each finger knuckle.

RIGHT: Soften the feet after a bath by massaging between the toes and then working around the tougher skin and heel areas. Finish with sweeping movements all over to stimulate the circulation.

PROBLEM ZONES

Hands and nails take some rough treatment with everyday chores. The ideal time for a manicure or pedicure is after soaking in a bath when nails and skin are softened, making it easy to clean around the nail bed and to clip uneven nails without snagging.

Fragile or flaky nails benefit from a rich, nourishing treatment: rub them with apricot kernel, wheatgerm or jojoba oil. Restore hands with a soothing, moisturizing mix of 15 ml (1 tbsp) sweet almond oil and 5 drops each of patchouli, lavender and lemon.

Feet are often neglected until they hurt. Polish hard skin around heels and soles with a handful of damp salt or use a pumice stone. While in the bath, bend one knee, grip the toes and then work with the fingers massaging in an upward direction, from the toes to the heels and up the calves in order to stimulate blood flow and relax tired feet. Massage a body oil into the feet after a bath, shower or pedicure.

For a deodorizing and soothing footbath add 3 drops each of cypress and lavender to a basin full of water. Chilblains can be treated with a massage blend of 3 drops of geranium and a drop each of lavender and rosemary in 15 ml (1 tbsp) sweet almond base oil.

with neroli, and peppermint has an affinity with melissa. Use a total of 6 drops in 20 ml (1½ tbsp) of base oils, with smaller quantities of rosemary (for example, 4 drops of rosemary to 6 drops of melissa). For fast relief add 4 drops to a handkerchief and inhale.

HEADACHES

Often one of the first signs of stress and a regular affliction for many people. Cold compresses of lavender or geranium across the forehead provide pleasant relief. Add 5 drops of one oil to a small bowl of cool or warm water, soak a cloth in the water, wring out and lay it across the forehead. To help a headache caused by tension in the neck, try a sandalwood compress across the neck. Scalp massage is soothing, or try the shiatsu headache relief steps (see page 318).

DEPRESSION

The blues can hit us all from time to time, as financial, emotional or work problems hang over like a dark cloud. In the long term, if problems are not resolved, depression lowers the immune system, leaving you prone to a spiral of worsening mental and physical health. Essential oils can work wonders in lifting the spirits to prevent this.

UPLIFTING OILS
Bergamot • Cypress • Lemongrass Rosemary • Sage

SOOTHING OILS
Chamomile • Geranium • Jasmine Lavender • Marjoram • Neroli Patchouli • Rose • Sandalwood Ylang-Ylang

Start off with three soothing oils, and then drop one of these in favour of an uplifting oil to give an element of stimulation, and eventually introduce two

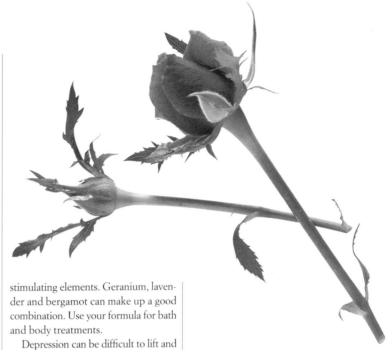

stimulating elements. Geranium, lavender and bergamot can make up a good combination. Use your formula for bath and body treatments.

Depression can be difficult to lift and if it persists you should consult a doctor or mental-health professional.

MENTAL FATIGUE

When you feel near to exhaustion or cannot concentrate on one thing at a time because problems seem to be crowding in on you, listen to your body's warning signals. Take time to unwind (try a bath with any of the soothing oils listed for depression), clear your head with a walk or deep-breathing exercises, and then revive yourself with oils such as eucalyptus and peppermint. Rosemary is helpful in concentrating the mind and stimulating the body so that you can continue to work if you feel you really cannot afford to take a break.

INSOMNIA

Sleeplessness is a common response to stress, as your mind and body refuse to let go enough to give you the rest that you need. Learning to relax has to be built into a daily pattern with a healthy diet, regular exercise, and a calming routine to wind down before bedtime. Try a milky drink or herbal tea last thing at night. Have a relaxing bath and massage, drawing on the sedative powers of up to three of the following oils:

Cedarwood • Chamomile Frankincense • Hyssop • Lavender Marjoram • Melissa • Neroli Orange • Patchouli • Rose • Sage Sandalwood • Ylang-Ylang

Breathing aromatic vapours in the bedroom helps to induce sleep:
❧ *Frankincense* is warming and relaxing, and encourages tranquillity. Use in a fragrancer.
❧ *Lavender*'s relaxing quality can be harnessed by dabbing 2 drops on the edge of your pillow.
❧ *Marjoram* has excellent soporific properties. Release in a light-bulb ring or fragrancer.
❧ *Neroli*'s wonderful floral fragrance is also sedative. Disperse unpleasant thoughts with 2 drops on the pillow or in a fragrancer.

HEADACHE RELIEF

Headaches and migraines are common symptoms of stress. Follow these simple shiatsu steps to sweep away the tension, relieve pain and clear the head. The sequence is quick and easy to administer; it can be used anywhere and friends and colleagues will be grateful for the relief of their pain. You can perform some of the steps on yourself, though the healing touch of another's hands is more effective.

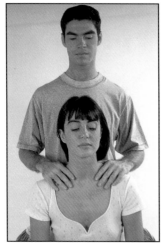

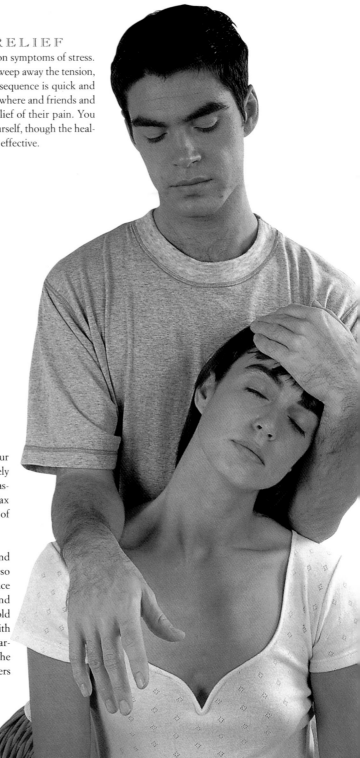

1 Establish communication with your partner by placing both hands loosely on either side of the neck. Gently massage the shoulders; this helps to relax the breathing and creates a feeling of well-being.

2 RIGHT: Tilt the head to the side and support with the palm of the hand so that the neck muscles can relax. Place the forearm across the shoulder and apply gentle downward pressure; hold for 5–10 seconds and then repeat with the other side. This movement is particularly good for opening the meridians running along the shoulders and neck.

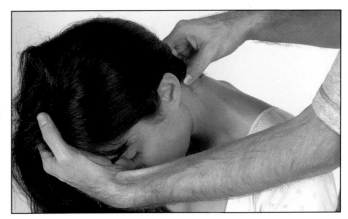

3 Supporting the head with the left hand, work with thumb and forefinger applying gentle pressure from the base of the neck to the nape. Hold at the nape of the neck for 5 seconds and then release the built-up tension.

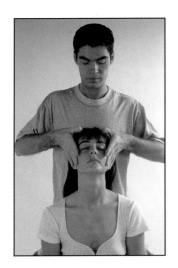

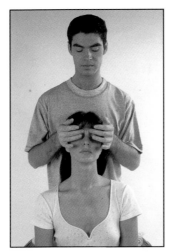

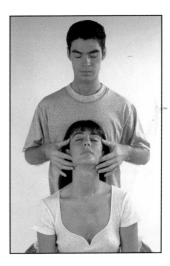

4 Tilt the head back slightly, supporting it on your chest. Place your thumbs on the temples with the fingers loosely resting on either side of the face. Gently rotate the thumbs in small forward movements.

5 Find the pressure points just above the inner corner of each eye. Apply gentle pressure with the middle fingers to help disperse the pain. Hold the pressure points for 5 seconds.

6 Position your thumbs on either side of the head just above the hairline – approximately 5 cm (2 in) apart – with palms pressed flat along the sides of the face. Press the thumbs evenly back along the top of the head.

A shiatsu treatment is usually very effective for relieving stress and headaches but if your headache persists, consult a doctor. Avoid the treatment during pregnancy.

LEARNING TO RELAX

❖═o═❖

R elaxation is a prescription for health. Along with a well-balanced diet, an exercise programme, and a positive attitude towards recognizing and coping with stress, relaxation will help you balance the body and mind, even when you are worried and under pressure.

Exercise combats stress. The physically fitter you are, the better the body and mind can cope. Even burning off steam without losing self-control can be beneficial: a competitive racket sport, thumping the pillow, or going for a long walk can all release built-up tensions. Times of stress and emotional upset can make the body cry out for certain foods. Resist chocolate, cakes, ice cream or addictive stimulants like caffeine. Feed the mind with a high intake of Vitamin C from fresh fruit and vegetables, in particular citrus, berry and tropical fruits, and all the B-complex vitamins.

WHOLE-BODY RELAXATION

Lie down straight with shoulders relaxed and even on the floor. Arms should be straight with elbows alongside the waist, palms turned upward. Relax your head and close the eyes. Breathe in deeply; allow your body to sink into the floor. Breathe out slowly; relax. Focus attention on your breathing; listen as you inhale and exhale and see how quiet the deep breathing can become.

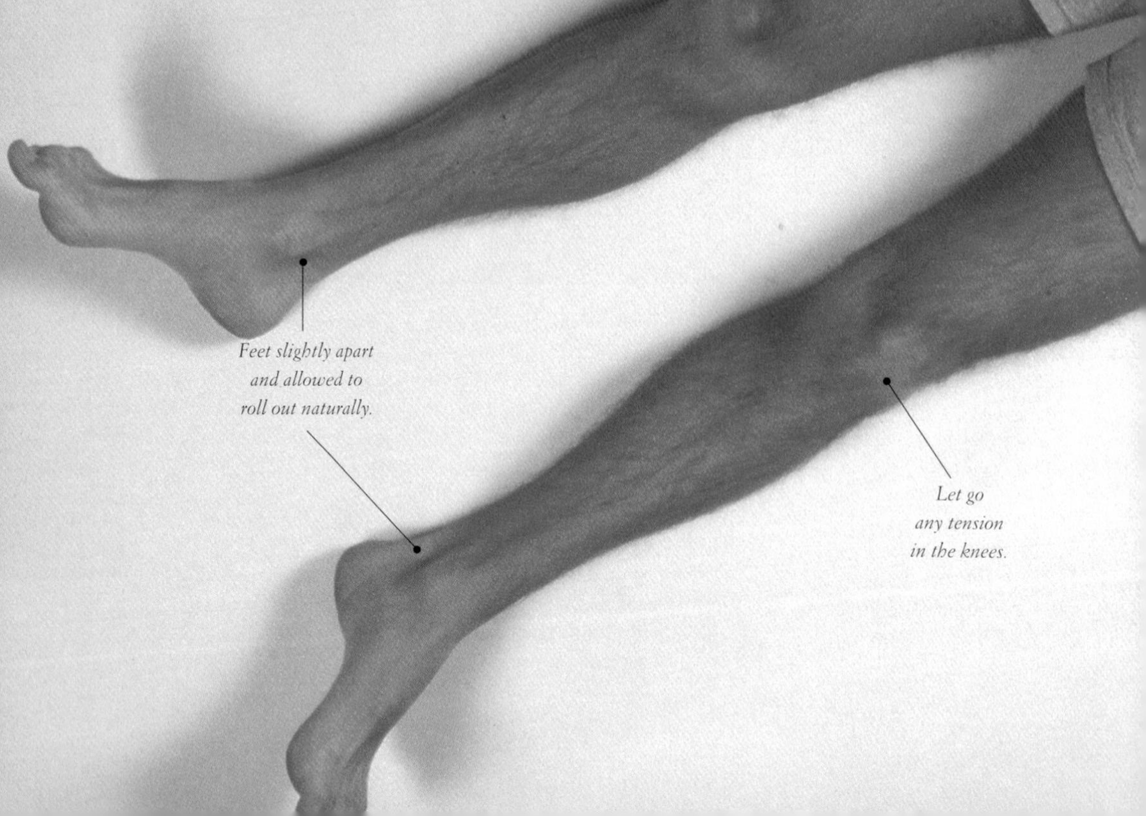

Focus on breathing in and out, slowly and evenly.

Feet slightly apart and allowed to roll out naturally.

Let go any tension in the knees.

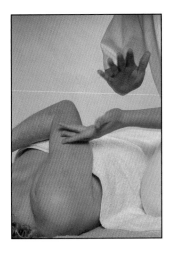

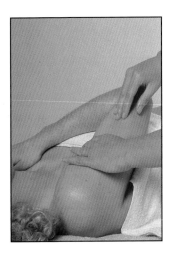

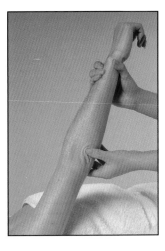

6 Bend your partner's arm and rest the right hand on the left shoulder. Using the outside edge of your hands, do some short, brisk hacking on the outer and under sides of the arm.

7 With your partner's arm still bent, firmly knead the muscles of the upper arm with your right hand, using the left hand to keep your partner's arm stable.

8 Holding the wrist for support with your right hand, work around the outside of the elbow with your fingers and thumb, using smooth circular movements and covering the area thoroughly. As the elbows can get dry you may need some more oil.

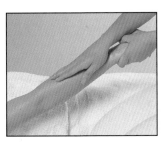

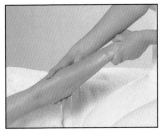

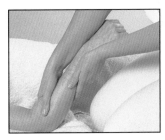

9 To encourage further relaxation, hold the wrist with the left hand and do some *effleurage* strokes up and down the top of the forearm. Keep the pressure fairly firm.

10 Repeat these *effleurage* strokes on the inside of the forearm.

11 Rest your partner's elbow back on the towel. Supporting the weight of the lower arm in your left hand, use your right hand to knead the inside of the forearm, starting from the wrist. When you reach the elbow glide back to the wrist to begin again. Repeat three times.

Finish the arm with a few *effleurage* strokes and then massage the hand and wrist (see the following pages) before moving on to the other arm.

HANDS AND WRISTS

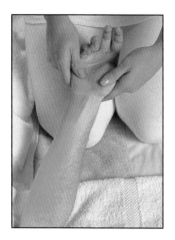

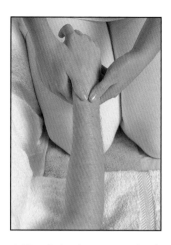

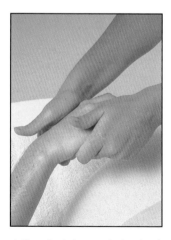

1 Support your partner's hand in both hands and gently use the thumbs to knead the palm. This should be a continuous, circular action, with the thumbs alternately applying pressure.

2 Rest your hands under your partner's wrist and use the thumbs to stroke outward around the wrist. Then work with the thumbs up the inner forearm toward the elbow, using circular movements.

3 Turn the hand over, supporting the wrist. Massage gently over the back of the wrist with your thumbs.

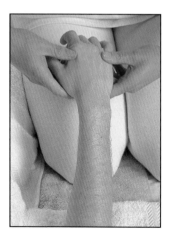

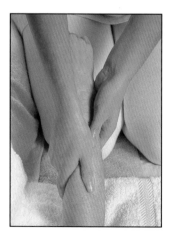

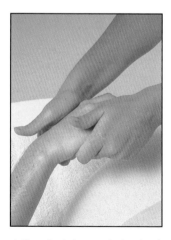

4 Stroke up in between the tendons on the back of the hand with your thumbs, from knuckles to wrist, using circles. Repeat twice between each tendon.

5 Sweep the hands alternately up from the wrist toward the elbow, applying a fairly firm pressure with the inside edge of the hands. Repeat several times.

6 Come back down to the hand and stretch the back of the hand, drawing your hands out toward the sides.

BACK

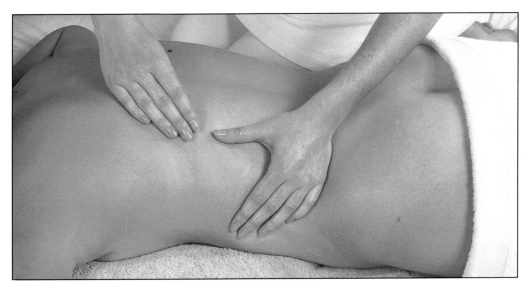

1 Kneeling to the right side of your partner, start to knead the far side of the back firmly with both hands, beginning at the outer sides of the waist. Pick up, roll and release the muscles, alternately pressing one hand toward another. Continue kneading up the back until you reach the shoulders.

Start again at the waist but this time come closer to the spine and repeat the line of kneading up the back.

Repeat the kneading on the near side of the back. You should be able to do this without moving your kneeling position.

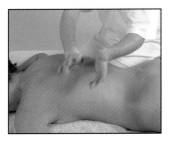 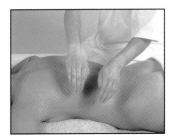 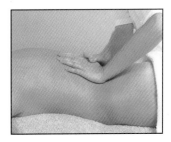

2 Using the outer edge of the hands, briskly and rhythmically hack from the lower back up to the shoulders, but avoid the bony shoulder blade. Try to visualize each side of the back divided into three sections, so you cover the whole back thoroughly.

3 Start cupping from the lower back up the back and across the shoulders. The action should be quick, with alternate hands striking the back briskly.

4 Repeat the *effleurage* strokes from the beginning of the sequence to soothe the back. Repeat several times.

SPINE

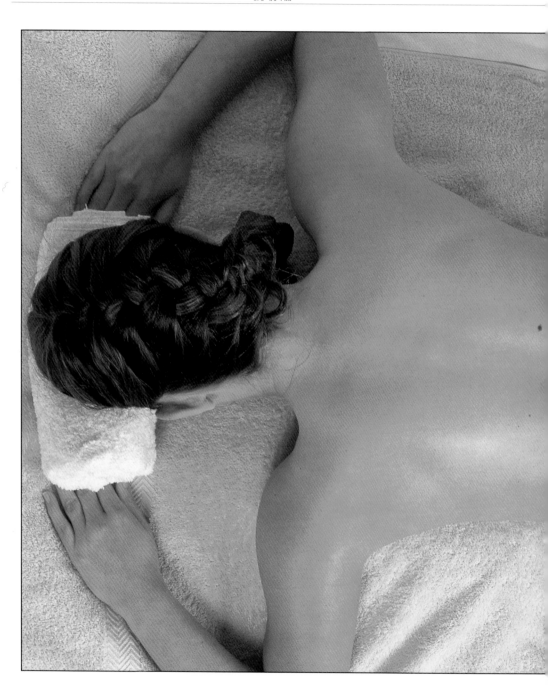

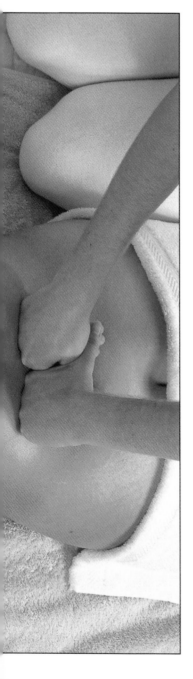

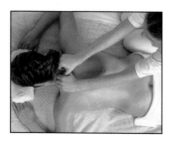

1 LEFT: With loose fists, and thumbs crossed for support, push the top of the hands up each side of the spine to the nape of the neck.

2 RIGHT: Uncurl the fingers when you get to the nape and sweep them back down the sides of the back. Repeat three times.

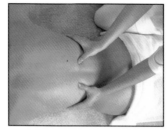

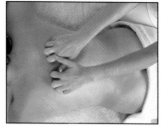

3 Starting at the lower back, place the thumbs on either side of the spine, resting your hands either side of the back. Rotate the thumbs in small circles, travelling up the sides of the spine until you reach the hairline. Use firm pressure. Reverse the movement, circling your thumbs back down each side of the spine.

4 Starting at the lower back, use loose knuckles, crossing your thumbs over each other for support, to work up either side of the spine and back down again. Repeat twice.

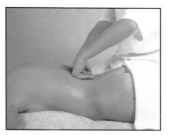

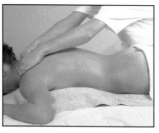

5 Using the backs of your hands and starting at the lower back, push up either side of the spine to just above the waistline. Then sweep your hands outward and back down around the hips. Repeat three times.

6 To finish the massage, repeat the *effleurage* strokes from the beginning of the sequence, starting at the lower back, up the back, around the shoulders and down again to the lower back, in a continuous sweeping movement.

SELF MASSAGE

⟡

A simple, effective self massage can do wonders to ease away tension and restore energy after a stressful, tiring day. After a shower or bath, massaging the body with lotions and oils is very relaxing and helps keep the skin in glowing condition. You can use self massage to target particular aches and pains or areas of tension, for relief just where you need it. The beauty of self massage is you can do it to suit your needs and moods at any time – to unwind in the evening or to energize yourself in the morning.

SHOULDERS

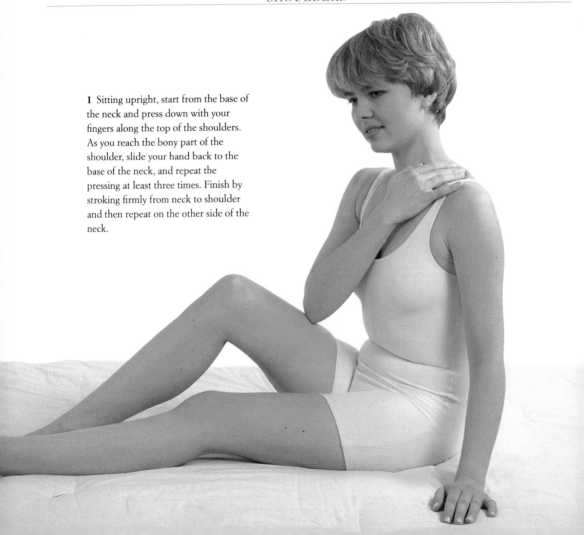

1 Sitting upright, start from the base of the neck and press down with your fingers along the top of the shoulders. As you reach the bony part of the shoulder, slide your hand back to the base of the neck, and repeat the pressing at least three times. Finish by stroking firmly from neck to shoulder and then repeat on the other side of the neck.

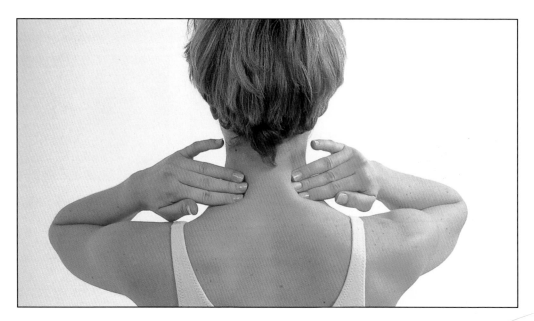

2 Use the fingertips of both hands to make small, circular movements, working up the back of the neck.

Gentle circular movements, where you can feel yourself easing muscular tightness, are better than direct, static pressures on this area. Continue up and around the base of the skull.

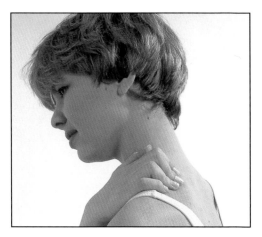

3 Knead each shoulder with a firm, squeezing action, rolling the flesh between your fingers and the ball of the hand. Repeat several times on each side.

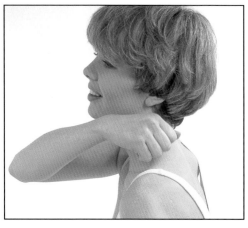

4 With your hand in a loose fist, pummel your shoulder lightly, keeping the wrist and elbow relaxed. Use light, springy movements to stimulate the area. Repeat on the other shoulder.

ARMS

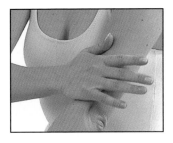

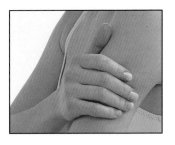

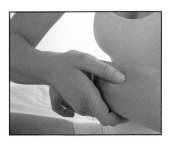

1 Stroke firmly up the arm from the wrist to the shoulder, returning with a lighter touch. Repeat the stroke several times on different parts of the arm.

2 Pressing your fingers toward the palm of the hand, knead up the arm from the elbow to the shoulder. Cover the area thoroughly, working right around the arm.

3 Starting from the wrist, knead up the forearm toward the elbow, this time using your thumb to make circular movements.

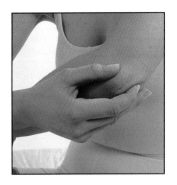

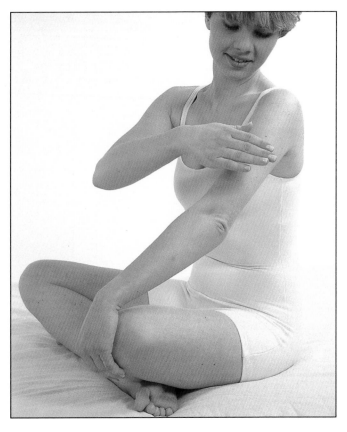

4 With thumb and fingers, make circular pressures around the elbow. First, work around the far side of the elbow with your working arm coming over the top of the arm you are massaging, then bend that arm up and work from the inside of your elbow. You may need more oil for dry elbows.

5 RIGHT: Gently but briskly pat your upper arm, or use some gentle cupping. Follow with some *effleurage* stroking up and down the whole arm again to finish. Work on the hand before massaging the other arm.

ANKLE STRAIN OR SPRAIN

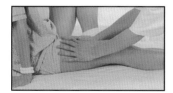 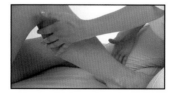 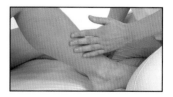

1 ABOVE and BELOW: Avoid working directly on the swollen area. Start with gentle *effleurage* strokes working from the knee toward the thigh. Massaging in the direction of the lymph nodes in the groin will help drain away the fluids that have accumulated around the joint. Lightly stroke back to the knee. Repeat several times.

2 Help your partner to bend the affected leg. Continue the *effleurage* strokes on the lower leg, this time working from the ankle to the knee, alternating your hands. Repeat several times, then gently squeeze the calves with one hand, with the other supporting the foot.

3 Concentrating on the ankle area, stroke extremely gently all around the ankle with short, upward movements. Check that this is not causing discomfort.

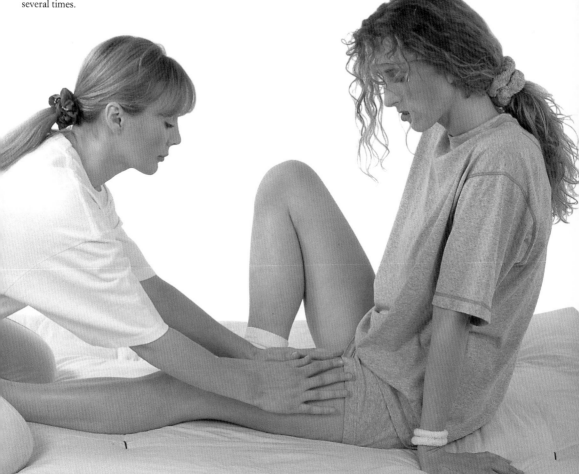

CALF CRAMP

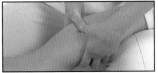

1 With your partner lying face down and the foot supported across your leg or a small pillow, gradually apply direct thumb pressure into the belly of the cramped calf muscle for 8–10 seconds.

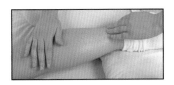

2 Do some *effleurage* strokes, working from ankle to thigh and back down again.

SELF-HELP STRETCH

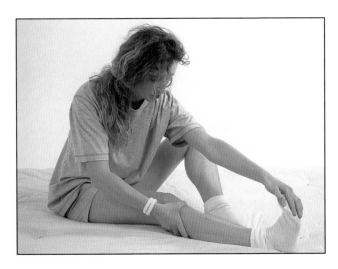

A good way of dealing with calf cramp is to sit down with the affected leg straight and stretch the toes toward you. Hold this position for 8 seconds and then release. Repeat a few times, until the spasm seems to be lessening. Then knead your calf muscle using firm pressure. When the muscle feels more relaxed switch to *effleurage* strokes, working up the leg.

HAMSTRING CRAMP

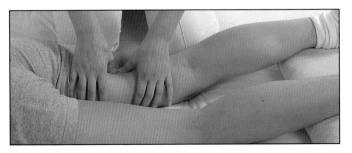

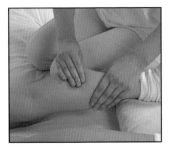

1 With your partner lying face down and the ankles raised on a small pillow or cushion, begin massaging up the back of the thigh using alternate hands in slow, rhythmical stroking movements.

Then apply static pressure to the middle of the thigh with the thumbs, holding for 8–10 seconds.

2 Firmly knead the calf muscle. Squeeze, press and release the muscle using one hand after the other. Finally, do some soothing *effleurage* strokes up from ankle to thigh and back down again.

HAMSTRING SELF-HELP STRETCH

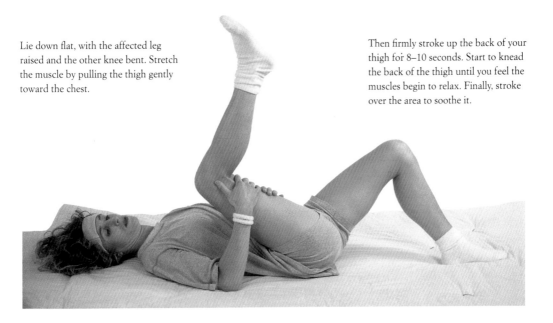

Lie down flat, with the affected leg raised and the other knee bent. Stretch the muscle by pulling the thigh gently toward the chest.

Then firmly stroke up the back of your thigh for 8–10 seconds. Start to knead the back of the thigh until you feel the muscles begin to relax. Finally, stroke over the area to soothe it.

TENNIS OR GOLFER'S ELBOW

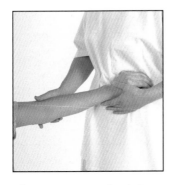

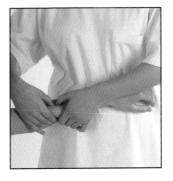

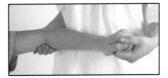

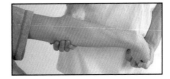

1 Support your partner's wrist in one hand and use soothing *effleurage* strokes along both sides of the arm, stroking from the wrist to the elbow and back again. Repeat several times.

2 Rest your partner's hand against your side. Continue working up from the wrist to the elbow and back, making small, circular movements with both thumbs, paying particular attention to the muscles in the forearm.

3, 4 Secure your partner's hand in yours, and with the other hand supporting the elbow, flex the elbow forward, bringing the hand back to give the tendons that attach to the bones a good stretch.

BABY MASSAGE

✦⇒◦⇐✦

A newborn baby instinctively responds to touch, and massage between mother and baby is a marvellous way of enhancing the natural bonding. All babies have this powerful sensitivity to being caressed and cuddled. Watch how a baby tightly curls its hands or toes as soon as something touches them.
There is no fixed sequence for massaging a baby. Keep the movements gentle and flowing. The simple action of gently stroking a baby will strengthen the natural bonding, and soothe and reassure the baby too. Massage has been shown to help calm difficult or colicky babies, and alleviate wind and other digestive problems. It may also build resistance to coughs and colds. Use a little light vegetable oil which is easily absorbed, such as sweet almond or sunflower, taking care to avoid the eyes.

GETTING COMFORTABLE

Lay the baby gently on the back on a warm, soft towel between your legs, or on your lap, whichever is most comfortable. Pour about 5 ml (1 tsp) sweet almond oil into a small dish. Make sure your hands are warm and that the room is quiet, very warm and there are no draughts. After a baby's bathtime is ideal.

WORKING ON BABY'S FRONT

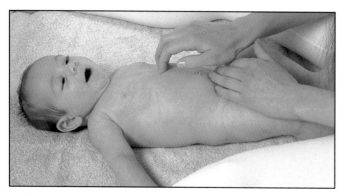

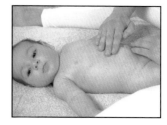

2 Keeping the pressure very light, smooth both hands over the abdomen in continuous, circular strokes, working up the baby's right side, across and down the baby's left side. Keep the movement continuous by lifting your left hand when your arms cross. Repeat these circular strokes several times.

1 Slowly and gently, smooth a little of the oil all over the front of the baby's body, shoulders to feet, avoiding the face. Lightly stroke down the chest and abdomen, with the tips of your fingers. This is a delightful stroke which can be used to calm a baby at anytime.

daily routines

The most surprising point about the Alexander technique is that it is not just for big, set piece movements such as lifting heavy weights, when doing it incorrectly can obviously lead to back problems. The technique even extends to the minutiae of life, routines that we completely take for granted, such as eating, drinking, and driving. If you had always wondered how they should be done, read on. These tips will make all the difference.

EATING AND DRINKING

If you are standing upright while you are drinking remember that you still need to be fully alert at all times. Therefore, make sure that you do not fix your gaze rigidly and thereby lose all communication and contact with the outside world. You also need to ensure that your head leads you away from your heels (see the section on Standing for further guidance). You will find that your shoulder girdle brings mobility to your arms, and that the pelvis provides stability which simultaneously facilitates mobility in your legs.

The very same principles also apply to eating. Whether you are going to eat something from your hand or use a fork, it is all too easy to forget your posture completely. Remember that you should not totally focus on the matter in hand, but that you must also consider your stance, alertness and poise.

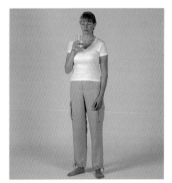

Avoid gripping or clutching your glass. Be aware of the connection with your arm, which links to your back and then into your heels. As you raise the cup to your lips, bring your weight back on to the heels, so as not to pull in your lower back. Also, bring the glass to the lips, rather than leaning down into it.

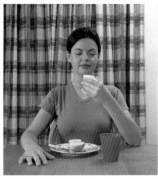

Take some time to consider how you are seated at the table and then bring the food up to your mouth, rather than the reverse. Your feet should be correctly positioned on the floor. You should also be aware of both your sitting bones, and how your back should be lengthening and widening. This position also aids digestion.

DRIVING

Most of the problems experienced by drivers are due to fixed postures, long journeys and poor seating support.

Too many people who spend huge amounts of time driving find themselves constricted by the position of the steering wheel and the pedals. Such a cramped environment is bound to lead to stress and strain on the back, and equally on the arms and legs.

When choosing a car take time to see whether the seat is firm and supportive. If you already own a car and it does not have a lumbar support adjustment, you can use a wedge-shaped cushion to give you adequate support in the lumbar area and the pelvis. It makes a vital difference.

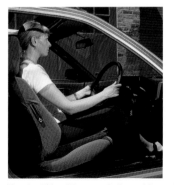

You should be able to reach the pedals quite easily. A wedge-shaped cushion is extremely useful to avoid a poor, slumping position.

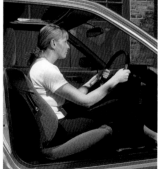

See how the model is badly collapsing forward, how the neck is being strained and the arms are rigidly tense. Such a position will cause lots of discomfort.

office work

Before reading it is important to spend some time considering exactly how you are going to sit in order to avoid badly slumping, which is very easy to do, especially in a big old comfortable armchair. Once you get drawn into what you are reading it is virtually certain that you will completely forget about your posture. It is vitally important that you do not end up creating all kinds of stresses and strains in your body.

READING AND WRITING

When you are sitting at your desk or at a table, it is important that you adjust your chair in such a way that your lower arms and hands can be placed on the surface of your table or desk at a right angle. If your chair is too close you are likely to end up lifting your shoulders to adjust your arms. If your chair is too high, you will probably find that you start slumping. You must also avoid crossing your legs, and do make sure that your feet remain comfortably flat on the floor.

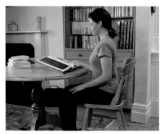

A useful trick when reading is to use a sloping board to avoid slumping over your desk or table.

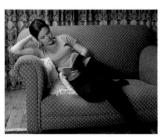

Note how the model is holding her body badly with her arm, and how her legs are folded, offering no support.

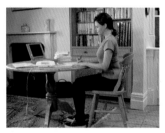

Keep the alignment between your head, your neck and your back.

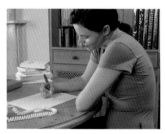

This model is firmly gripping the pen, causing tension in her wrist and hand.

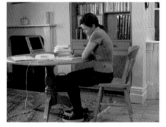

Here the model is tensing her wrist, hand and arm, restricting her movement.

DESKWORK

An increasing number of people are complaining of neck and shoulder tension, wrist problems and back pain resulting from their working environment. Some cases are directly linked to badly designed furniture, awkward or unfavourable sitting positions and immobility. In other instances, although chairs and work surfaces are good, the posture is poor. You must therefore remember your primary directions: the head, neck and back should be aligned, and the head should be lengthening away from the sitting bones.

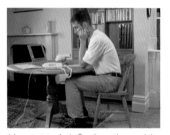

How not to do it. See how the model is slumping badly, causing unnecessary tension in the spine, so weakening the muscles surrounding the torso.

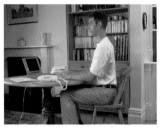

Here the spine is correctly aligned, and the head is poised gracefully above the neck. The feet are well placed on the floor, nicely apart.

office equipment

The office is not what it used to be. It now offers amazing improvements in high-tech equipment, but also plenty of opportunities for repetitive strain injury, aching backs and tense necks. The temptation is to spend far too long in one awkward position. So always be aware of what you are doing, how long it will take, and the best position you need to adopt. Such awareness makes all the difference between a good and bad day.

MOBILE PHONE USE

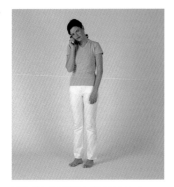

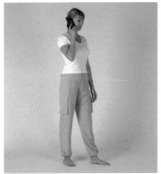

Observe Yourself When the Telephone Rings

Do you snatch and grab it? Or do you try to give yourself some time before you pick up the receiver? Next time the telephone rings, stop and go over your primary directions. Make sure that you bring the receiver up to your ear rather than suddenly leaning down towards it, thus compromising your position.

Here the model is pulling her head down wrongly towards her mobile phone to talk, and slouching.

In this example the model has maintained her balance throughout her body. She looks poised and relaxed.

WORKING AT A COMPUTER

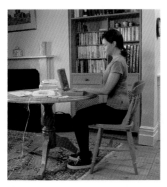

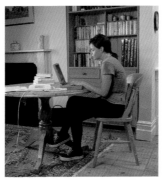

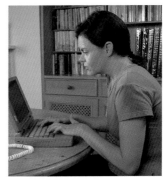

If you are working at a computer or portable computer, use your eyes to look down towards it. Avoid lurching at the neck as you will lose the correct alignment with your back.

Here the model badly collapses over her computer. She has lost the correct alignment between her hands, her wrists and her lower arms. Her shoulders are far too hunched.

Here the model is incorrectly holding in her wrist, arms and shoulders, causing unnecessary strain and discomfort. She will soon feel very uncomfortable, and have to adopt a new position.

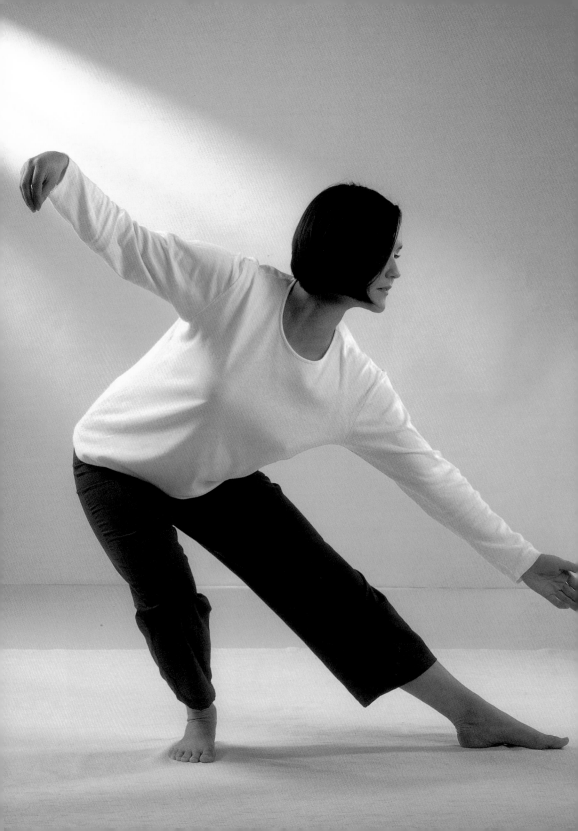

t'ai chi

t'ai chi
t'ai chi

T'ai chi ch'uan is an ancient form of slow, graceful and rhythmic exercise which originated in China, where it is still extremely popular, often being performed in public parks in the fresh morning air. It has its roots in Taoist philosophy. The movements of the t'ai chi form gently tone and strengthen the organs and muscles, improve circulation and posture, and relax both mind and body. Its name translates as "supreme ultimate fist", but this is not its true meaning. "Strength within softness", "poetry in motion" and "moving harmony" all come closer to expressing the spirit of t'ai chi.

T'ai chi has been variously described as a system of health, medicine, physical co-ordination, relaxation, self-defence and consciousness raising, as well as a means of exercise and self-development. It is all these things. The style shown here is the Yang-style short form, as developed by Professor Cheng Man-Ch'ing, which is the one most practised in the West.

Unlike the "hard" martial arts which rely on force and speed, t'ai chi is "soft" or "internal". Its emphasis lies in the yielding aspect of nature when overcoming the hard – like the waterfall which eventually wears away the rock beneath. It teaches patience and relaxation, and fosters an understanding of the co-ordination of mind, body and spirit. It is the perfect antidote to the stresses and strains of today's modern lifestyles.

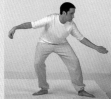

t'ai chi for health or self defence If you

simply want to go out and strike a pose, jumping about like Bruce Lee, t'ai chi is not for you.

It is a very serious, highly regarded ancient technique that has two major qualities. It improves

your health, and teaches you how to overcome stronger hostile forces when you are under

attack. The most amazing part of t'ai chi is the way its movements are almost balletic.

The Benefits of T'ai Chi

Although t'ai chi can eventually be used in self-defence, and most classes do incorporate some of its practical applications, it is initially practised mainly for its health-giving benefits. It is particularly useful for increasing alertness and body awareness, and for developing concentration and sensitivity. It helps with balance and posture, and enhances a sense of "groundedness". However, all the postures can also be used when defending yourself against an attack by an opponent. Its gentleness and subtlety do not preclude its use as a very effective form of self-defence.

It is not easy to separate the physical and mental aspects of t'ai chi, as they are closely interrelated. In Chinese medicine, the interdependence of mind, body and spirit is seen as integral to well-being.

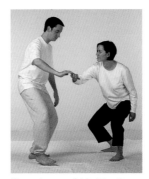

The ancient art of t'ai chi instills enormous grace and confidence.

The Theory of T'ai Chi

Like music, t'ai chi cannot be appreciated purely on an intellectual level. It also has an enormous spiritual side, and when you watch any highly experienced t'ai chi practitioners you will see how they are almost in a kind of trance, in a separate world where they cannot be touched. Correctly done, it is quite hypnotic.

For now, we must look at some of the concepts that are fundamental to the martial arts, as well as to medicine and philosophy. Although these disciplines are all treated quite separately by those in the West, they are all inseparable in the Eastern view. From thousands of years of close observation of patterns of energy, the Chinese successfully evolved a way of life that actually ropes all three ingredients together.

Chi

Chi is the prime driving force of human life, the spark behind thought, creativity and growth which maintains and nurtures us. It can be felt as movement of energy in the body, like the ceaseless flow of an electrical current. Chi flows through the body along channels called meridians.

The Tan Tien

The Chi is stored in the Tan Tien. This is an area about the size of a golf ball, located four finger-widths below the navel, and about one-third of the way from the front to the back of the body. It is the centre of gravity of the body, and in t'ai chi all movement emanates from it. Try to let the breath and the mind sink to the Tan Tien.

Yin and Yang

Yin and Yang describe the complementary yet opposing forces of nature. Their relationship has a harmony and balance: both Yin and Yang are necessary, are constantly moving and balancing each other, and this interaction creates Chi. The Chinese observed that when the balance of Yin and Yang is disrupted so too will be the body's Chi, leading to ill health.

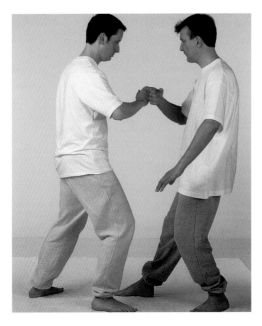

One of the key requirements for t'ai chi is excellent balance.

warm-up exercises

Perform these exercises slowly and gently, with the mind and the breath focused in the Tan Tien. Notice any differences between the right and left sides of your body, and between the upper and lower parts. The object is gradually to enter the world of t'ai chi, and to warm up all your muscles so that you do not get any strains. The more you warm up, the better your technique will be. The movements will flow like a stream.

CIRCLING HANDS

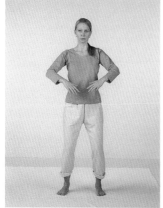

1 Inhale and allow both hands to float upwards a comfortable distance in front of your body, palms facing downwards.

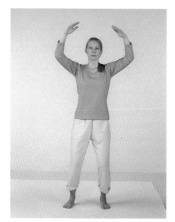

2 As your hands rise above your head, relax the wrists and begin to open the palms outwards. Begin to exhale.

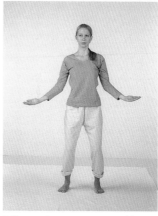

3 Open out your arms to your sides. Draw your hands inwards at the bottom of the circle and smoothly begin again.

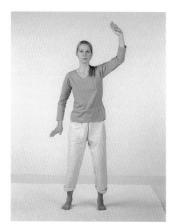

4 Inhale as your palms, facing upwards, float in front of your body. Exhale and push your right hand down by your hip and your left hand up by your temple.

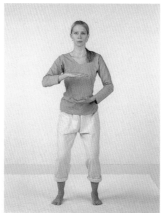

5 Breathe in again, relax your palms which now turn to face each other and begin moving them towards each other in front of your body.

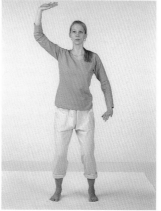

6 Repeat step 4 in reverse as you exhale. Breathe in again and bring your hands in front of your body in a mirror image of Step 5.

SHAKING OUT SHOULDERS, ARMS AND HANDS

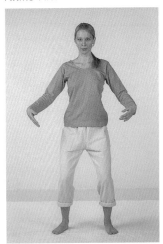

I Gently shake out any tension in your wrists and hands. Gradually work up to include your shoulders. This exercise is especially useful before, during and after long periods at a keyboard, or repetitive work with the hands.

LOOSENING SHOULDERS

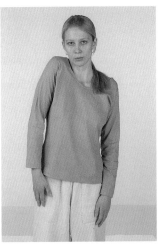

I Make increasing circles with one shoulder. Change direction and decrease the size of the circles. Repeat for the other shoulder. Rotate your shoulders alternately.

ROTATING WAIST

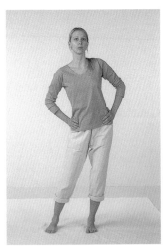

I Place both hands lightly on your hips. Keeping your head up, begin by spiralling your hips slowly outwards, feeling for any restriction, tightness or lack of ease. Change direction and spiral back in slowly.

KNEE ROTATIONS

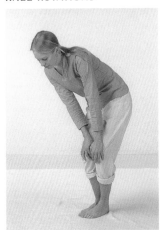

I Bring your feet together and place your palms lightly on your upper kneecaps. Feel the Chi from your palms radiating deep into your knee joints. Circle your knees clockwise several times, then change direction.

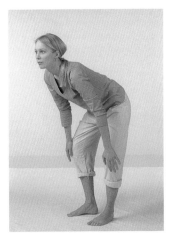

2 Keep your legs and hands in the same position. Rotate your knees in opposite directions — one circles clockwise while the other circles anti-clockwise (counter-clockwise). Change the direction of each knee and repeat the rotations.

CALF STRETCH

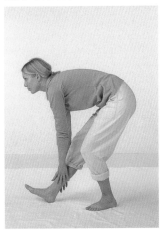

I Step forward with your right foot. Keeping the heel on the floor, pull up your toes towards the knee. Drop your body forward, keeping your right leg straight. Hold for a few breaths and release. Repeat for the other leg.

PLAY GUITAR. BRUSH LEFT KNEE AND PUSH

This posture is also known as "Strumming the Lute".

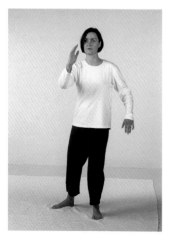

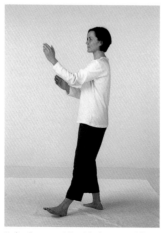

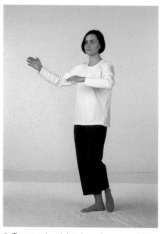

5 Take a shoulder-width step with your left foot, heel first. Move 70% of your weight into your left leg as your left hand brushes down across it. Meanwhile, your right hand follows a concave curve into the centre to finish by the mouth.

1 As all your weight sinks into your left leg, adjust the "empty" right foot by drawing it slightly nearer the left foot, toe first. Bring your weight into the right foot. Your left leg and arm float up simultaneously – imagine a thread connecting them.

2 Turn to the right, dropping your right hand down while your left hand follows the movement of your waist to the centre of your chest, palm facing down. As your waist returns to the front, your right hand comes to shoulder height.

STEP FORWARD, DEFLECT, INTERCEPT AND PUNCH

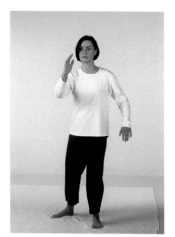

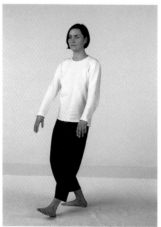

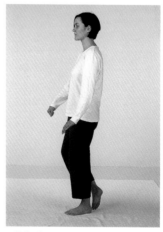

3 Take a shoulder-width step with your left foot, heel first. Move 70% of your weight into your left leg as your left hand brushes down across it. Your right hand follows a curve ending by your mouth.

1 Turn your waist 45° to the left and sink all your weight into your right foot. As the weight shifts back, lift the toes of your left foot and pivot 45° on the heel. Bring your hands down by your left leg.

2 Shift all your weight into your left leg. Form a loose fist with your right hand, but check that the fingers are not wrapped around the thumb. The right toes are behind the left heel.

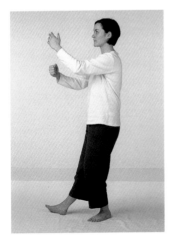

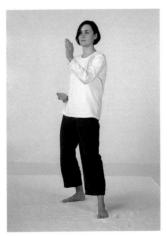

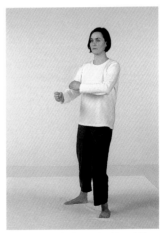

3 Arc both of your hands and your right foot simultaneously towards the centre line, as your waist turns around to the right. The right foot now lands "empty", in line with the left instep. Check that your position is correct. Note that your left thumb should roughly be in line with your left eye.

4 Continue to turn your waist to the right, bringing the right fist palm upwards to rest on the right hip. You should now commence transferring all your weight on to your right foot. Your eyes should skim across the tops of your left fingers.

5 Place your left foot a shoulder width from the right foot. Shift 70% of your weight to your left leg and bring your right fist forward as if to punch, rotating it through a quarter turn in a corkscrew motion. Then bring your left arm across your body, with the palm facing your inner right elbow.

WITHDRAW AND PUSH. CROSSING HANDS

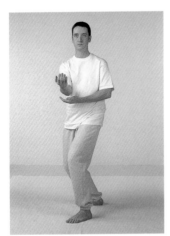

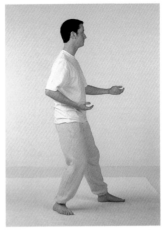

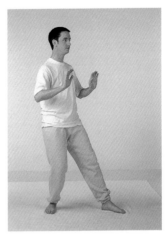

1 As you turn your waist to the left, your right arm follows your body to an angle of 45° and the fist opens up. Meanwhile, cup your left hand gracefully a couple of inches under your right elbow, as if supporting it.

2 Draw your right arm across your left palm as your weight sinks into your right foot, and your waist turns to the right.

3 Bring your waist back to the centre and turn both palms to face the front.

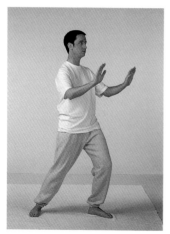

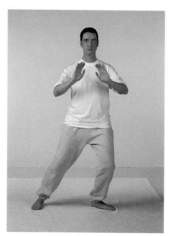

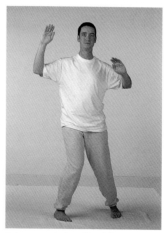

4 Move your weight forward 70% on to your left leg. Your hands remain at shoulder width and shoulder height.

5 Turn your waist to the right and simultaneously sink all your weight into your left leg. Draw your hands in towards your chest in a softly inverted "V" shape, as if holding the top of a ball.

6 As your whole weight shifts into your right leg, turn your waist to the right. Your left toes turn with your waist and your right hand travels out both diagonally and upwards.

EMBRACE TIGER, RETURN TO MOUNTAIN

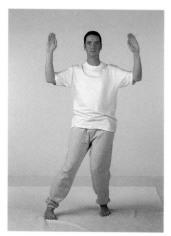

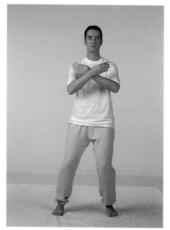

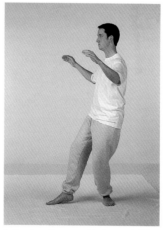

7 Sink all your weight back into your left leg. Your left hand now travels out diagonally. Though the position might seem slightly awkward and lopsided, it actually flows naturally into the final step.

8 Finally, bring your right foot shoulder-width away from and parallel to the left, but maintain your weight 70% in the left leg. Both hands circle down and up, stopping opposite your chest, palms facing the body. The wrists are touching, with the right wrist outside the left one. Hold this stance for a few seconds.

1 Keeping all your weight in your left leg, turn your waist to the right. Open your hands outwards. Step diagonally back with your right foot. Move your weight 70% on to your right foot. As your waist completes its turn, move your left hand so that the fingertips are in line with your left shoulder, palm facing forward.

ROLL BACK, PRESS AND PUSH: SINGLE WHIP

PUNCH UNDER ELBOW

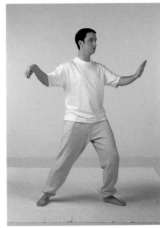

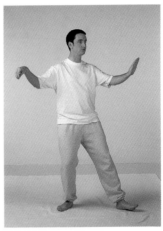

2 As you turn your waist slightly to the right, allow your left hand to come across so that the fingertips point to your right elbow. Meanwhile, your right hand travels upwards so that the fingertips point heavenward.

1 Now repeat the sequence in "Roll Back, Press and Push". This time, perform this section from one diagonal corner to the other rather than from one side to the other. This picture shows your position at the end of the sequence.

1 Sink all your weight back on to your right foot. Turn your waist 45° to the left, lifting the left toes and letting your left foot and both arms pivot 45° to the left.

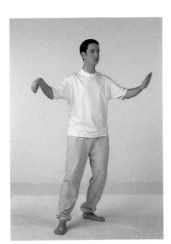

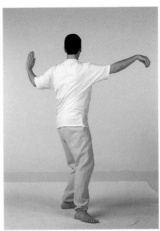

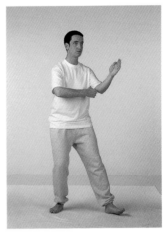

2 Lower your left foot, gradually shifting your weight forward into it. When all your weight is on your left foot, step forward with your right foot so that the heel is in line with your left instep.

3 Rotate your upper body 90° to the left. Your arms follow this waist movement, so that the hook (your right hand) is now out in front level with your right shoulder, and your left hand is level with your face at 90° to the front. Your weight is in your left leg.

4 Transfer all your weight to your right leg, turning your waist to the right and letting your left hand move down, then up, until the fingers are in line with your left shoulder. Your left arm and leg move around simultaneously. Rest your left heel on the ground without any weight.

FAIR LADY WEAVES SHUTTLES (RIGHT AND LEFT)

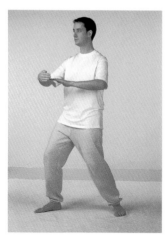

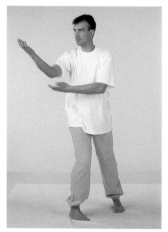

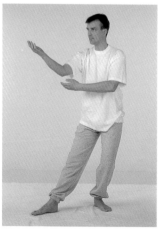

3 Step through at shoulder width with your "empty" right foot. As you transfer 70% of your weight into it, your right hand comes up into a ward-off position opposite your chest, with the left fingertips now pointing towards the right palm, left palm downwards. Repeat "Roll Back, Press and Push" and "Single Whip".

1 Transfer your weight to your right leg as you turn your waist to the right, and turn the "empty" left toes through 90°. Bring your left hand across your body and under your elbow. Open the hook of your right hand and lower the right arm, palm turning to face upwards.

2 Sink your weight back into your left leg, turn your waist further to the right and turn out your right foot so the heel is in line with the left instep.

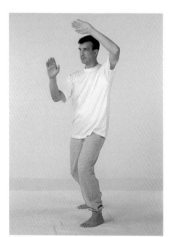

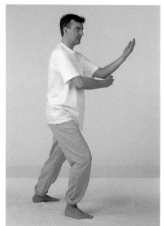

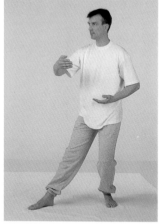

3 Sink your weight into your right leg, drawing your left arm across your right palm, and step at shoulder width to the left corner with your left foot. As you shift your weight forward into your left leg, turn both palms outwards.

4 Transfer your weight into your right foot and turn your waist and left foot to the right as far as possible (135°). Turn your palms to face your body, the right palm by the left elbow.

5 Sink your weight back into your left leg and draw your left arm across your right palm.

FAIR LADY WEAVES SHUTTLES (RIGHT AND LEFT)

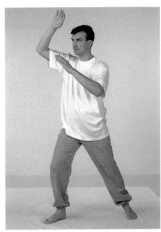

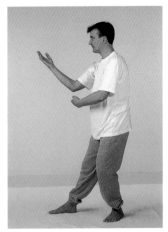

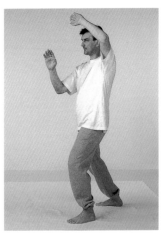

6 Turn a further 135° right, to the corner. Step to shoulder width with your right foot, and shift 70% of your weight into it, pushing towards the centre of your mouth with your left hand. Bring the right hand up to guard your forehead, palm facing diagonally.

1 Turn to the left, sinking all your weight into your left leg. Pick up your right foot and draw it in. Transfer all your weight to your right foot, then step to the left (45°) with your left foot. Turn your palms in and draw your right arm across the left palm, left arm in a ward-off position.

2 Your left hand then moves up and turns outwards by your head, while the fingers of your right hand come into the centre in line with your mouth. Now repeat the postures described in Steps 4, 5 and 6 of the previous exercise.

WARD OFF LEFT. WARD OFF RIGHT. ROLL BACK, PRESS AND PUSH. SINGLE WHIP

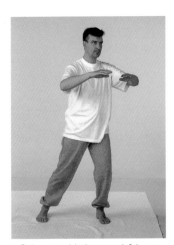

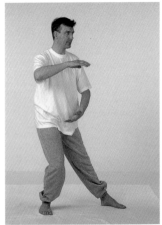

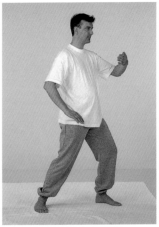

1 Sink your weight into your left leg as your waist turns to the left. Both arms come round with the movement of your waist, the left hand lower than the right. The right toes come round to the front.

2 Sink your weight into your right leg as your left hand presses down, palm facing downwards. Take a shoulder-width step with your left foot.

3 Transfer your weight 70% into your left foot. Your left hand comes up in front of your chest. Your right hand floats outside your right thigh. Repeat previous step.

SQUATTING SINGLE WHIP. STEP FORWARD FOR SEVEN STARS   RIDE TIGER

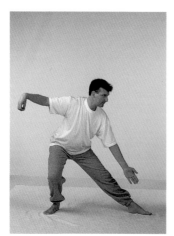

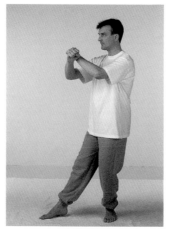

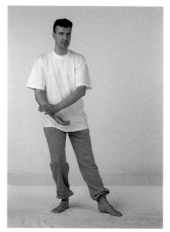

1 Repeat the postures described in Steps 1, 2 and 3 of "Golden Rooster Stands on One Leg (Left). Squatting Single Whip", ending by brushing open the left knee.

2 Transfer all your weight into your left leg. The right hand hook opens and the hand descends, then comes up in front of your neck, where it forms a loose fist. At the same time, your left hand rises up to form a loose fist, and connects at the wrist inside your right hand. Move your right toes forward to touch the ground without any weight whatsoever.

1 Keep your weight in your left leg and step back with your right foot, toes touching the ground first. Sink your weight into it and turn your waist to the right. The fists open and then move down by your right hip, with the wrists still connected.

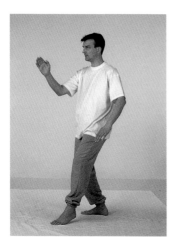

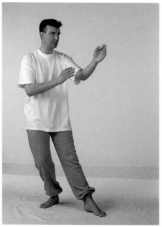

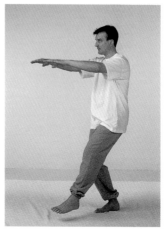

2 Pick up your left leg as your waist turns right, then place your toes down as your waist turns back to the left. Your right hand comes round to the front, fingertips level with your right ear, and your left hand rests by your left thigh.

3 Pick up your left toes, turn your waist to the left corner and place the toes down empty of any weight. Your right palm faces your inner left elbow. Your left hand is at the height of your left shoulder, elbow relaxed.

4 Lift your left toes and swing your waist clockwise, pivoting on the ball of your right foot. Your arms swing to the right with the movement of your waist.

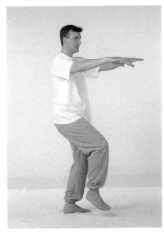

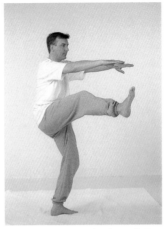

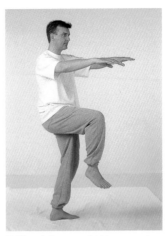

5 Drop your left foot and transfer all your weight into it straight away. Look closely at the photograph above to check how you should be standing.

6 When your arms and waist reach the front (the arms at shoulder height and shoulder width with the palms facing downwards), your right foot lifts up and circles clockwise.

7 After circling, your right leg comes to rest with the upper leg parallel to the ground and the foot comfortably relaxed. Your left leg is bent while the arms are still pointing ahead.

BEND BOW TO SHOOT TIGER. STEP FORWARD, DEFLECT DOWN, INTERCEPT AND PUNCH

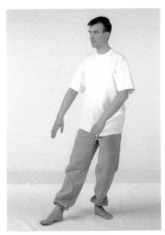

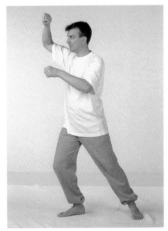

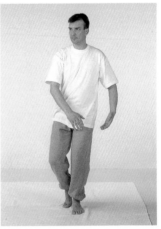

1 Turn your waist to the right. Your arms follow your waist, dropping down parallel, and your right foot is placed facing the right corner.

2 As your waist turns to the right, shift the weight into your right leg and circle your arms round to the right. As your waist turns back to the left, raise your arms and circle round with the waist. Form loose fists. Bring the right hand up to the right of your forehead, knuckles facing the right eyebrow. The left hand is at shoulder height.

3 Sink your weight into your left leg and pick up your right foot, placing the toes by your left heel. Open the left fist as your arms move across your body following the waist movement.

WITHDRAW AND PUSH.
CROSSING HANDS. CONCLUSION.

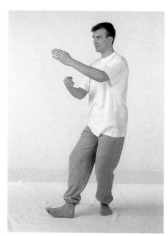

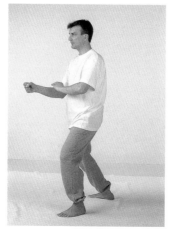

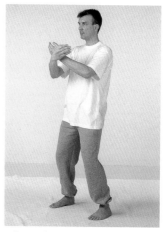

4 Both hands and your right foot simultaneously arc in towards the centre line, as your waist turns to the right. The right foot lands "empty", completely in line with the left instep.

5 Continue to turn your waist, bringing the right fist palm upwards to rest on your right hip and shifting your weight to the right foot. Step through at shoulder width with your left foot. Shift 70% of your weight to the left and bring your right fist forward to punch in a corkscrew. Your left arm comes across your body.

1 Repeat the postures described in "Withdraw and Push. Crossing Hands". Ensure your weight is 70% in your left leg when crossing hands.

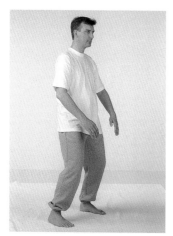

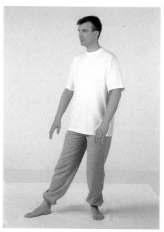

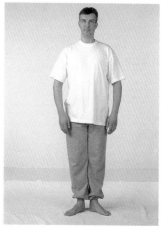

2 From crossing the hands, turn both palms down to face the ground as your body now rises up.

3 Bring all your weight into your left leg, turn your waist to the right and pivot on your left heel, turning the foot out to an angle of 45°.

4 Move all your weight into your right leg. Step in with your left foot so that the feet make a right angle. Bring half your weight to the left foot. Rest your arms and hands by your side with shoulders relaxed. You may now begin again.

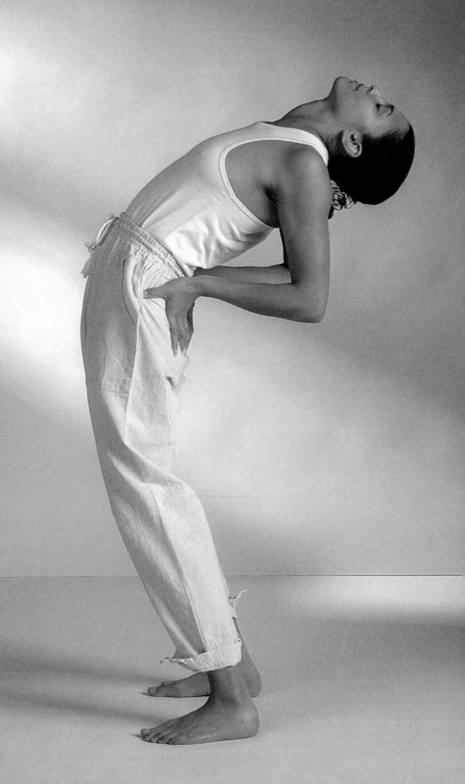

yoga stretches
yoga stretches

yoga stretches

Have you ever watched a cat waking up? More often than not, it will give an exaggerated yawn, then arch its back until stretched to its limit, before loosely letting go and gracefully moving off on its way. Have you ever stopped to wonder why it makes these movements? The cat knows instinctively the value of stretching in maintaining flexibility and improving circulation to the muscles; you too can become stronger and more flexible with regular stretching exercises.

Most of us tend to hold in patterns of tension arising from everyday cares and worries, bad posture, lack of exercise and so on. These patterns make us feel stiff and unbending, and directly interfere with our movements. Inflexibility within our bodies can in turn affect mental flexibility, and we can become stuck in thought as well as in action. Regular stretching exercises not only free our bodies, allowing us to move easily, but can also help us to think and act without being so restricted. They are excellent improvers. In fact, by stretching muscles, ligaments and tendons, we make them much more efficient and stronger. The lengthening actions also help us to stand and walk taller, and even with added grace. The joints are better supported and are more able to go through their full range of movements, while the muscles are better nourished from the increased blood supply. The stretches give you that extra edge.

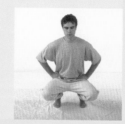

warm-up exercises
As any athlete will tell you, before starting to do any serious stretching or exercise, such as tennis, it is important that you first do some gentle warm-up exercises. They ensure that your muscles are nicely warmed and loosened, and will help to prevent any sudden strain or injury. The best thing is they only take a few minutes, and they can also be practised at any time if you are feeling stiff and need to loosen up.

SHRUGGING SHOULDERS

ARM CIRCLING

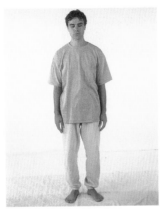

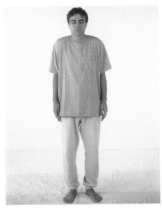

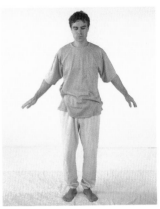

1 Stand upright with your feet slightly apart and your shoulders relaxed.

2 Lift your shoulders up as high as they will go, then let them fall down again. Stay relaxed and repeat a few times.

1 Wheel your arms around from the shoulders in slow, large circles.

SQUATS

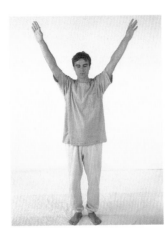

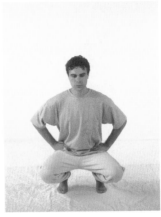

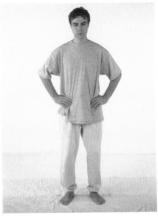

2 Do this a few times going backwards, then repeat circling your arms forwards.

1 Stand with your feet slightly apart, hands on hips. Go slowly into a squat.

2 Slowly return to a standing position, then repeat. Your back should be upright.

meditation

meditation
meditation
meditation

Meditation has been in use from the beginning of time:
people have always sought inner quiet and physical
relaxation, whether for reasons connected with the spirit,
self-realization or health. You do not have to be a physical
contortionist to achieve and enjoy the benefits of meditation
at both physical and mental levels.

What, then, is meditation? It has been described as just
sitting and relaxing. Many people find that their lives are so
full of the demands of work, family, friends and organized
leisure pursuits that they have no time to "stand and stare".
Many are so caught up in planning and working towards the
future that they take little pleasure from the here and now. In
their bustle to "get on" they miss out on the simple pleasures
of life. But beauty and joy are there to be seen and
experienced, even in industrial cities.

The benefits of meditation come from regular use. If you
are under stress, you may find that meditating twice daily will
be effective in restoring composure. Make a time and space
you can call your own, and use breathing and relaxation
exercises to ease yourself into the meditative state. The more
you practise meditation the less time you
will need to spend on these, but they
remain useful in calming and preparing you.
Allow at least 10 minutes, ideally 20, for
meditation in each session.

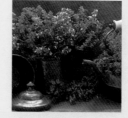

the benefits of meditation

Human beings were never designed to cope with the high-pressure demands of life in the 21st century; life when you are constantly in demand, having to make vital decisions at breakneck speed right through the day, and even during the night. You might say it cannot be done, but it can, with help. Knowing how as well as when to switch off makes all the difference, and even scientists now agree.

PSYCHO-PHYSICAL LINKS

A period of meditation can often lead to a feeling of being refreshed, with a more positive attitude and a general feeling of well-being. Things that had been bothering you may now be seen in a new and more helpful way. You gain a different, wider perspective on things and feel very much more in control.

These beneficial reactions have been well known for years, but only in recent times has anyone found a physiological explanation. Detailed, extensive knowledge of brain scans and even brain wave patterns has given extraordinary new information about what is commonly called the "alpha state".

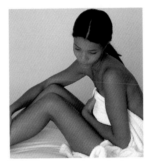

Mind and body work together in meditation to promote health and well-being in the whole person.

Endorphin Release

When we are truly relaxed, both mentally and physically, there are changes in the brain wave pattern until it is predominantly located and fixed within the alpha state. Within this particular state the brain triggers chemicals known as endorphins. It is in fact this chemical trigger that has the benefits that are experienced as a feeling of well-being. Indeed, endorphins have frequently been called "nature's very own special opiates", and these good feelings can easily linger for some time after the meditation has ended, the length of time varying considerably. There is also a real physical benefit, as these endorphins boost and recharge the immune system, helping you to fight off all kinds of infections.

Meditation and Work

The tensions of modern working practices often mean that people are so bound up in meeting all the vigorous demands placed upon them that they maintain a high level of mental and physical activity right through the day. This frequently means that they are not only cutting off their extremely important emotional responses and their enjoyment of the simple things in life, but they are also pushing their physical and mental health right to the very limit. Much has now been written about the management of stress, and the significant need for periods of mental and physical relaxation during the working day.

The 20-minute Rule

One writer, Ernest Rossi, has formulated the 20-minute rule which is based on the theory of ultradian rhythms. Ultradian rhythms are biorhythms that the body works through during each day – a little like hyperbolic curves of energy which repeat every 90 to 120 minutes. Naturally, it would be best to work only at peak performance times, but this is just not possible. However, timing work breaks to coincide with the mind/body slow-down pattern every 90 minutes does ensure maximum productivity and restricts the potential build-up of stress.

Rossi suggested the pattern of working for 90 minutes and then taking a brief 20-minute break. He himself usually lies down and meditates during this period because it is the best form of total mental and physical relaxation, and is good preparation for returning to optimum mental processing.

It is important that these breaks take place every 90 minutes or so, and in such a way as to completely change the mind/body state. Ideally, you should stop all work activity and experience a change of physical status (standing rather than sitting, looking into the distance rather than close up, for example) and mental focus. A 20-minute meditation is ideal and the benefits will be felt immediately. On returning to work after the 20 minutes, you will see things afresh and deal with them more efficiently, as you are ready to climb to peak performance on the biorhythmic curve. The feeling of well-being lasts into the next 90-minute period.

To be at your best for meetings ensure you take regular breaks.

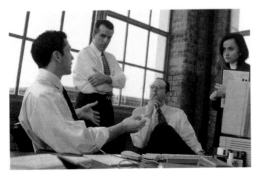

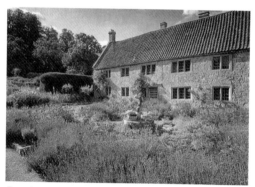

Try to imagine your perfect country house.

A GUIDED VISIT TO A COUNTRY HOUSE

Imagine that you are visiting a beautiful country house ... a really beautiful old country house or a stately home with magnificent sweeping lawns on a warm, sunny, summer's afternoon. You are standing on the staircase that leads into the entrance hall, one of those wide ceremonial types of staircase. And as you look down across the entrance hall you can just glimpse, through the open doors opposite, a gravel drive, and the sunlight on the gravel. It is a beautiful, sunny, summer's afternoon and there is no one around to trouble or bother you as you stand alone on that staircase ...

Now you are moving down the last ten steps to the hallway, relaxing more and more with each step down.

10 Taking one step down, relaxing and letting go ...
9 Taking another step down, feeling at ease ...
8 Becoming more relaxed, letting go even more ...
7 Just drifting deeper ... and deeper ... everything is getting darker and darker, and even deeper down still ...

6 Becoming calmer ... and calmer ... even calmer still ...
5 Continuing to relax, continuing to let go and feeling good ...
4 Relaxing even more ... letting go even more ...
3 Sinking deeper ... drifting even further into this welcoming, relaxed state ...
2 Enjoying those good feelings, all those feelings of inner peace and relaxation ...
1 Nearly all the way down now, feeling very good ... beautifully relaxed ... and **0**.

You are wandering across that hallway now, towards the open doors and the gardens beyond, soaking up the atmosphere of peace and permanence in that lovely old building. You wander out through the doors and down the stone steps outside ... and find yourself standing on the gravel drive outside, a wide gravel drive that leads down to the entrance gates.

As you stand there you notice the lush green lawns, so flat and well-clipped ... and there are shrubs and trees, different shades of green and brown against a clear, blue sky ... and you can feel the warmth of the sun on your head and shoulders as you enjoy this beautiful summer's afternoon in this lovely old garden ... There are flowerbeds with their splashes of colour so carefully arranged and neatly tended. And there's no one else about ... nobody needing anything, nobody wanting anything and nobody expecting anything from you, so you can enjoy the peace and serenity and solitude of this afternoon in this beautiful garden that's been so well looked after for so many, many years.

A little way down on the right-hand side of the driveway, you notice an ornamental fish pond. So you decide to wander down and have a look at those fish. Sometimes they seem almost to disappear behind the weed and shadows, but always they reappear, with their scales catching the sunlight, red, gold, silver or black. And as you watch those fish your mind becomes even more deeply relaxed ...

THE WELL

This continues from the previous visualization of the beautiful country house and is intended to take you to even deeper levels of meditation.

... As you watch those fish you notice that the centre of the pond is very deep. It could be the top of a disused well. You take from your pocket a silver-coloured coin, and toss that coin so that it lands over the centre of the pond, and then you watch as it swings down through the water. The ripples drift to the edges of the pond, but you just watch that coin as it sinks deeper and deeper through that clear water; sometimes it seems to disappear as it turns on edge, at other times a face of the coin catches the sunlight and it flashes through the water ... sinking, drifting deeper and deeper, twisting and turning as it makes its way down ... Finally it rests at the bottom lying on a cushion of soft brown mud, a silver coin in that still, clean water on its own cushion of mud ... And you feel as still as that coin, as still and cool and motionless as that water, enjoying that feeling of inner peace and stillness.

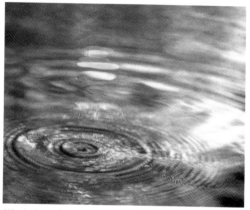

Watch the ripples as the coin lands in the very centre of the pond. Look even more closely as it tumbles down through the water ...

enjoyment and achievement

The mind and the body are so completely interlinked that if we keep physically fit we are also mentally alert. The one boosts the other, but it also works the other way around. If we really utilize our mental capacities we can affect and improve our physical health and performance. So it is up to you to make sure that these twin forces keep functioning at full power. Do not let either slip.

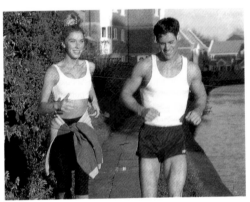

A well-tuned lively body keeps you feeling well and alert.

THE BODY/MIND LINK

Regularly say to yourself ...

- I feel safe, happy and content in the knowledge that my body is constantly renewing itself. It is alive and well.
- It feels marvellous to know that every damaged cell is replaced by a healthy one.
- My immune system is strong and fights off any infections easily.
- My mind and my body are working in harmony to keep me healthy, well and alert.

Now, imagine yourself lying or sitting comfortably. As you see yourself there you notice a healing glow of coloured light surrounding your body, but not touching it. Let that colour become stronger, until it has a very clear pure colour, which is the colour of healing for you.

Now, as you watch, that healing, coloured light begins to flow into the top of your head. You can see it slowly draining into all parts of the head, face, ears, and starts its journey down through the neck and shoulders, into the tops of the arms ... It continues to flow down through the arms and the chest area, that healing, coloured light, penetrating all the muscles and organs ... even as you watch you can also feel a healing warmth coming into your body ... NOW ... as it flows down into the stomach area, the back, right the way down to the base of the spine. Then you can allow the light to disperse again and gradually return to your normal wakeful state, knowing that in those areas that need it, the healing process will continue.

STRESS REDUCTION

Stress is a factor in everyone's life and can even be a major motivator in some circumstances. Meditation can be a great help in coping with it, and combined with visualization, it can change your whole response to stressful demands. Keep saying ...

- I enjoy solving problems.
- I work well under pressure.
- I am a calm, methodical and efficient worker.
- I love that feeling of having achieved so much in a day.
- I enjoy being calm when others around me are not.

Imagine yourself in a situation that has in the past caused stress. Picture the situation, and the other people involved ... See yourself there ... and notice a slight shimmer of light between yourself and those other people ... a sort of bubble around you ... a protective bubble that reflects any negative feelings back to them ... leaving you able to get on with your tasks ... your life, with an inner strength and calmness that surprises even you. A protective, invisible bubble surrounds you at all times. It will only allow those feelings that are positive and helpful to you to pass through for you to enjoy and build upon. Others may catch stress from each other ... negativity, too, can be infectious ... but you are protected ... you continue to keep things in perspective ... and to deal with things calmly and methodically. You are able to see the way forward clearly ... solve problems ... find ways around difficulties ... by using your own inner resources and strengths, born of experience. In you alone lies the secret of success. You can and you will succeed.

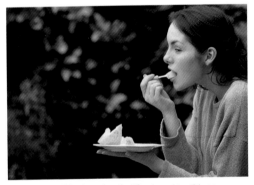

Imagine yourself leading a healthy lifestyle and it will happen.

LIVING NOW

Although we cannot change the past, we can learn from it and build up a range of skills and useful insights from it. The future is that unknown world of possibilities and opportunities before us – but all that we can truly have any effect upon is the present. Keep saying to yourself …

- I have learned a great deal from the past.
- The future is an exciting range of opportunities.
- I enjoy laying good foundations NOW on which to build a better future.

Imagine yourself standing on a pathway. As you look around the left, right and above is brilliantly illuminated, and sounds are amazingly clear. As you check over your shoulder you notice the path behind is unclear. You hear a clock chime in the distance and take a step forward. You notice the slightest of noises, movements or shifts of light, and take pleasure even in the pure sound of silence, too. You can hear that same clock ticking now, and with each tick you can take a small step forward, effortlessly, along the path, and that illumination and awareness moves with you. At any fork in the path you can make decisions easily as you are truly involved in the moment, rather than looking over your shoulder at what might have been, or staring blindly into the future at what might happen. You enjoy being in the brilliantly illuminated, acute awareness of sound, hearing, feeling, taste and smell that is NOW.

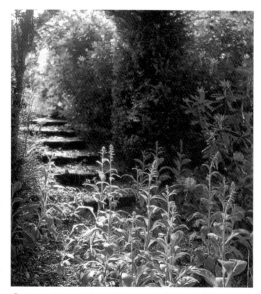

For a complete experience, be more acutely aware of shapes and textures as well as sounds, colours and scents.

GOAL ACHIEVEMENT

A goal, in all areas of life, is vitally important in order to focus your attention and inner resources. A goal provides a sense of direction and ultimately the joy of achievement. Without it you might flounder, so keep saying to yourself …

- I direct my energies to achieve my goals.
- I enjoy directing my energies positively.
- I know where I am going and how I am getting there.
- Step by step I am moving in the right direction.
- I have the ability, I have the determination, I shall succeed.

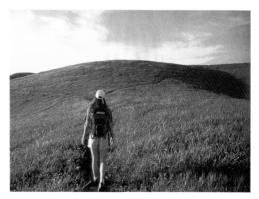

Keep your eyes firmly fixed on your goal and you will achieve it.

Be aware of the different areas of your life: work, social, leisure activities, emotional and spiritual. Select one of these for this exercise … and be aware of what you want to happen in that area of your life, what you want to achieve … Make it realistic and clear in your mind. It may be useful to write it down and describe it fully before beginning this visualization.

While in the meditative state, imagine yourself having achieved that goal, imagine yourself there, in that situation. Surround yourself with all the things or people that indicate that you have achieved that goal. Be as specific as you can … be aware of all the senses … what are you seeing … hearing … touching or sensing … smelling … tasting. Be there … make it real … be specific … about colours … temperatures … lighting, to make it more and more real in your mind.

Now, from where you are at that moment of achieving that goal … look back … as if along a path, a pathway of time … to where you were … and notice the different stages of change … of movement towards achieving that goal … along the way … along that path … the different actions you have taken … the contacts you have made … and the people involved. Be aware of all the stages along the way … and as you return to the here and now … you remain in touch with the feelings that will make it all worthwhile … and you feel more and more determined to take one step at a time … make one change at a time … along that path to the successful achievement of your goal. And as you return from the meditative state so you are more determined to be successful in the achievement of your goal.

General Fitness

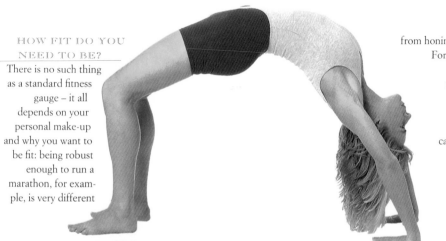

Fitness is the key to a healthy mind and body. It is based on stamina, strength, and suppleness – the three "S"s; better shape and self-esteem are two extra "S" bonuses. Being fit does not merely improve your physical prowess and grace, it also makes you feel better overall. But although we are more health-conscious about our diet nowadays, regular exercise is still not a part of most people's daily lives. Surveys always draw the same conclusion as to the reasons for this: lack of time, energy, interest, and confidence. Becoming fit is neither as difficult nor as time-consuming as it may appear to be: you can get fit – and get a better body into the bargain – more quickly, easily and enjoyably than you may think.

HOW FIT DO YOU NEED TO BE?

There is no such thing as a standard fitness gauge – it all depends on your personal make-up and why you want to be fit: being robust enough to run a marathon, for example, is very different from honing the three "S"s. For exercise to be of any help to you, though, it should boost your metabolism and improve your cardiovascular and respiratory systems.

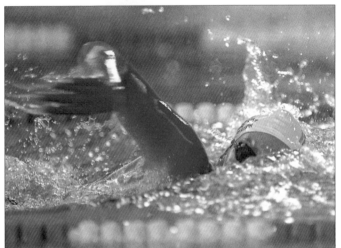

Swimming is an excellent way of keeping the whole body in good physical condition when done regularly and conscientiously.

WHY BOTHER WITH FITNESS?

Are you tired of running out of puff, being out of shape or always feeling under the weather? Do you often get colds, or suffer from pre-menstrual syndrome (PMS), stress, or sleepless nights? These are just a handful of the signs that could manifest themselves when you are unfit.

So exercise is worth the effort, because when you are fitter, problems such as these may ease or disappear.

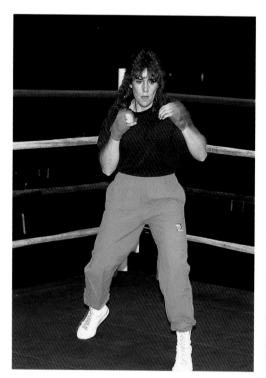

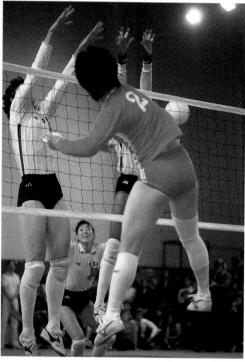

Women are increasingly attracted to strenuous sports such as boxing that until recently were considered to be solely a male preserve.

Competitive team sports such as volleyball not only provide an opportunity to improve physical fitness, they are also highly enjoyable.

YOUR GOAL

Finding a goal to inspire you is the secret of success. Set the deadline and stick to it. Depending on what you want to achieve, a three-week plan is ideal because it is not too long and if you persevere (take it week by week or day by day – whichever you find easiest), you will see results. Be realistic: if your goals are too high you are likely to fail: if they are too low, you will not have enough of a challenge.

Goals will inspire you, but speedy results are the key to keeping up regular exercise – it is natural to want to see rewards for all your hard work – although it is advisable to build up a pattern gradually. The minimum amount of exercise you need to do to improve your personal fitness is 20 minutes, three times a week – the "3 × 20" maxim. This means three bouts of exercise vigorous enough to make you fairly breathless (but not gasping for breath). So if you do the general fitness exercises outlined in this book three times a week for 20 minutes you will get fitter. If you want to see fast results, though, you need to add extra activities – such as a couple of games of tennis, swimming, or brisk walking – to your exercise quota, so that you are actually exercising six days a week.

Taking part in a team sport once a week is a good idea: not only will it make you fitter, slimmer, and happier, the competitive spirit will also strengthen your resolve. Some sports need special skills, but you do not have to be an athlete to do most of them.

CAUTION
Before taking up any form of rigorous exercise or training, you should consult your doctor – especially if any of the following conditions apply to you:

❧ diabetes or epilepsy
❧ over 35 years of age with a long history of inactivity
❧ cardiovascular or respiratory problems
❧ severe illness and ensuing medication
❧ chronic joint or back problems
❧ obesity
❧ pregnancy
❧ heavy drinking or smoking

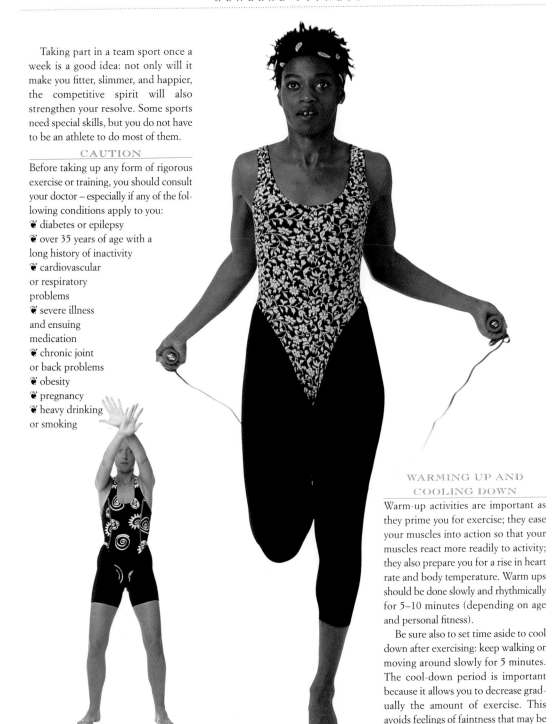

WARMING UP AND COOLING DOWN
Warm-up activities are important as they prime you for exercise; they ease your muscles into action so that your muscles react more readily to activity; they also prepare you for a rise in heart rate and body temperature. Warm ups should be done slowly and rhythmically for 5–10 minutes (depending on age and personal fitness).

Be sure also to set time aside to cool down after exercising: keep walking or moving around slowly for 5 minutes. The cool-down period is important because it allows you to decrease gradually the amount of exercise. This avoids feelings of faintness that may be caused by the pooling of blood below the waist that occurs during vigorous exercise.

YOUR PULSE RATE

Monitoring your pulse rate allows you to keep a check on whether you are exercising adequately. The maximum heart rate for an adult is roughly 220 beats per minute minus your age in years. The ideal heart rate during exercise is in a target zone of 65–80 per cent of this figure. The aim of exercise is to get your heart rate to within a certain range. These are the ideal exercise heart rates for the different ages:

Age	Pulse Range
20+	130–160
30+	124–152
40+	117–144

To find out your active pulse rate per minute, rest two fingers lightly on your pulse immediately after exercising, count the beats for 10 seconds and multiply by 6.

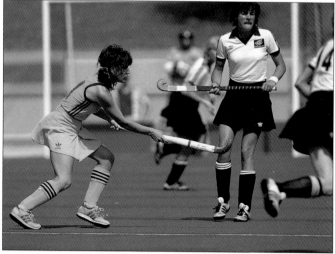

Hockey is a demanding sport that strengthens the legs, is beneficial to the heart and lungs, and significantly improves co-ordination.

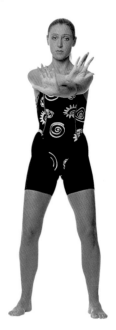

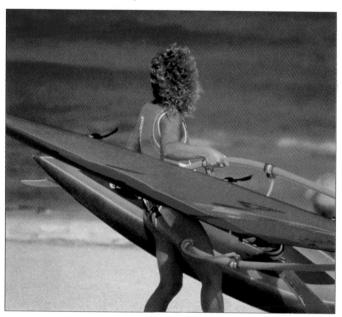

A good many water sports demand strength, stamina, and a fine sense of balance. Wind surfing is no exception to the rule.

EXERCISES FOR GENERAL FITNESS

This exercise routine helps to improve over-all fitness and should take you roughly 30 minutes to complete. Aim to do it three times a week and try to do extra aerobic exercise – such as swimming, walking or cycling – on the other days (aerobic exercises include any activity that can be done rhythmically and continually and that boosts the efficient uptake of oxygen). To warm up your muscles before exercising, either spend 2 minutes running up and down the stairs, walking briskly, cycling, or doing the special warm-up exercises outlined below.

WARM-UP EXERCISE A

1 Stand upright with your feet apart and in line with your shoulders, with your arms hanging loosely at your sides and your shoulders down.

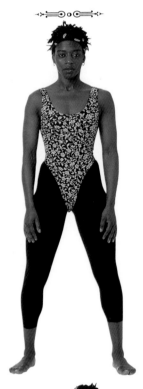

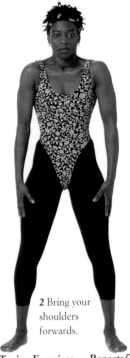

2 Bring your shoulders forwards.

❦ If you feel any pain – or experience anything other than the normal sensation of muscle fatigue – stop exercising. Always work out at your own pace; and skip exercise if you are ill.

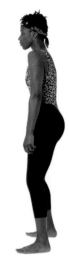

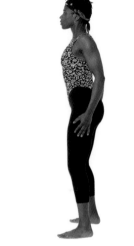

3 Raise them up high.

4 Move them back as far as possible, then back to the start position.

Toning Exercises	Repeats/Time Allowance
Warm-ups	5 minutes
Press-ups	10 repeats
Lying Flies	10 repeats
Reverse curls	10 repeats
Sit-ups	10 repeats
Squats	10 repeats
Cool Downs	3–5 minutes
Aerobic Exercise	20–30 minutes

The recommended 10 repeats are for beginners – you should aim to repeat each exercise 15 times. Start by doing this set of exercises twice a week, work up to three times a week and combine it with some other form of exercise – ideally aerobics – for the time suggested above.

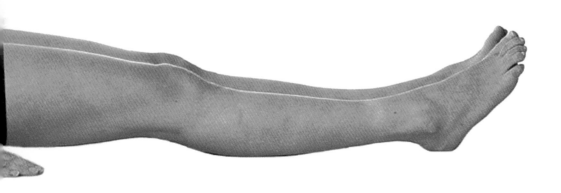

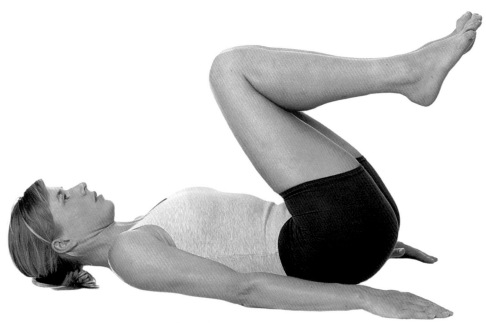

3 Breathe in and, keeping your spine pressed into the floor, pull in your abdominal muscles while at the same time curling up your coccyx (tail bone) to bring your knees closer to your chest. Keep your feet relaxed throughout. Lower your body to the starting position, exhaling as you go down.

SPORTS ACTIVITIES

❧

Team sports and work-outs at the gym are not only fun, they also give you the chance to add to your exercise quota for the week, and therefore reach your self-improvement goals that much faster. The benefits of taking part in specific sports and of working out are given here.

BADMINTON:

Aerobic; improves joint flexibility, stamina, leg and shoulder tone and strength; 30–40 minutes continuous play burns up around 200–800 calories.

GOLF:

Improves arm, shoulder and leg tone, and strength (you walk four to five miles when you do a round of golf).

JOGGING:

Aerobic, improves stamina, leg strength and tone; an hour's jogging burns up 200–350 calories. If you think that jogging or running will suit your new active way of life, take the standard precautions before you start: check with your doctor and, as with all aerobic exercise, increase the pace gradually; always wear the right trainers (and support bandages if your joints are weak).

TENNIS:

Aerobic; boosts stamina and suppleness; strengthens and tones your shoulders, forearms, calves and thighs; play energetically (ideally twice a week) for an hour and you will burn up around 300–400 calories.

BRISK WALKING:

Aerobic; strengthens and tones your legs.

CYCLING:

Aerobic; builds stamina; tones your legs.

SKIPPING:

Aerobic; boosts stamina, strength and leg tone. Start by doing 3 skipping sets for 30 seconds a time with a 5-minute break after each set; build up to skipping for 2 minutes with a 10-minute break and also increase the repetitions.

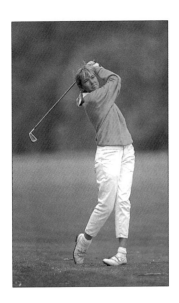

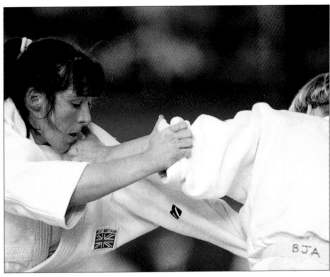

Golf is a sport that particularly benefits shoulders, arms, and legs. Playing a round involves a good deal of walking.

Judo is a body contact sport and one of the major martial arts. It requires a good deal of strength, agility, and physical courage.

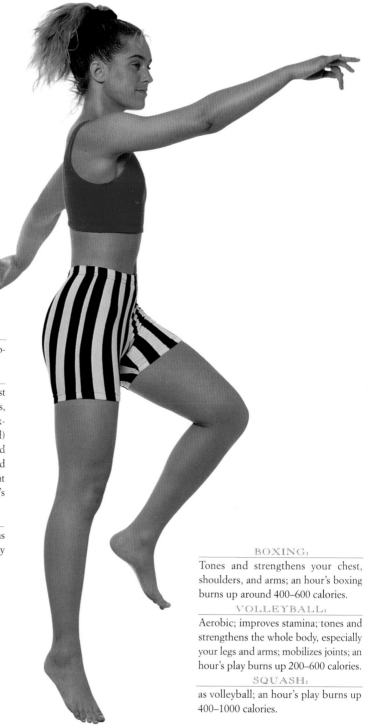

GYM-BASED BENEFITS
Aerobics: classes combine exercise with constant movement; they are fast fat-burners and ideal if you are after quick results.
Circuit, cross, resistance, or weight training: aerobic; increase stamina and strength; an hour of circuit training burns up between 350–550 calories.
Step classes: aerobic; improves stamina; tones and strengthens your lower torso; an hour-long class burns up between 500–800 calories.
Yoga: improves posture; tones, strengthens, and relaxes the body; loosens joints; an hour of yoga burns up about 200 calories.

REBOUNDING:
Aerobic; bounding on a mini trampoline is a fun way to get fit at home.

SWIMMING:
Aerobic; swimming is one of the fastest (and best) ways to boost overall fitness, muscle tone, joint flexibility, and relaxation. Do 4 lengths of a 25 m (25 yd) pool, rest for a minute and build endurance by reducing rest time and increasing swim time; within a fortnight you will be noticeably fitter; an hour's breaststroke burns 500–800 calories.

FOOTBALL:
Aerobic; improves stamina; strengthens and tones your legs; an hour's play burns up around 250–1000 calories.

HELP FOR PMS
Exercise is the last thing you feel like doing when you are premenstrual. But if you do push yourself now, you will relieve the symptoms. If you cannot face an aerobics class, go for a swim; this will ease pre-menstrual cramp and put you in a better mood.

BOXING:
Tones and strengthens your chest, shoulders, and arms; an hour's boxing burns up around 400–600 calories.

VOLLEYBALL:
Aerobic; improves stamina; tones and strengthens the whole body, especially your legs and arms; mobilizes joints; an hour's play burns up 200–600 calories.

SQUASH:
as volleyball; an hour's play burns up 400–1000 calories.

BODY SHAPE

The shape of your body is unique: it is important to remember this because the basic skeletal and muscular form that you inherit is unchangeable. Features such as your height, foot size, shoulder width and the length and shape of your legs, nose, fingers and toes combine to produce a whole. Each person is an individual, with characteristics particular to their genetic make-up.

BODY BRACKETS

Although we come in a variety of shapes and sizes, the human body is cast from three basic moulds. Often, features from two or three of these body types are jumbled with our individual characteristics, but it is the more dominant features that slot us into one of the following groups: ectomorphs; mesomorphs, and endomorphs.

Ectomorphs are usually small- and slender-framed with long limbs, narrow shoulders, hips and joints. They have little muscle or body fat. Mesomorphs have medium to large – but compact – frames with broader shoulders, pelvic girdle and well-developed muscles. Endomorphs are naturally curvaceous, with more body fat than muscle, wider hips, shorter limbs and a lower centre of gravity than the other two body types.

SELF-IMAGE

If you are a bit on the tubby side, it can be annoying to hear someone who you think is poker-thin whining about being overweight. But there is logic behind this that stems from self-image. Very few of us actually see ourselves as we really are. We tend to misjudge our bodies with sweeping claims to fatness, even when we have only a spot of excess flab around our midriff to show for it. And although it sounds amazing, the way we behave in everyday life (and think others see us) often tallies with our self-image. It is a vicious circle: we think that we do not measure up to the standard beauty ideal so our self-esteem dips, often so low that we feel that we will never have a better body. This in turn causes self-confidence to plummet further, we feel even worse, and so the vicious circle continues.

Taking control of your self-image brings enormous bonuses. And the faster you can do this, the greater the rewards, as speedy results boost your confidence more quickly. But before you undertake a scheme to get into better shape, you must work on your positive thinking: realize your potential by deciding on (and accepting) your body model, then use this as your goal. Forget conventional beauty ideals – you do not have to have mile-long legs to have a dynamite figure; what you already have – your basic shape – is great. It just needs perfecting, and that is something that everyone can do with determination.

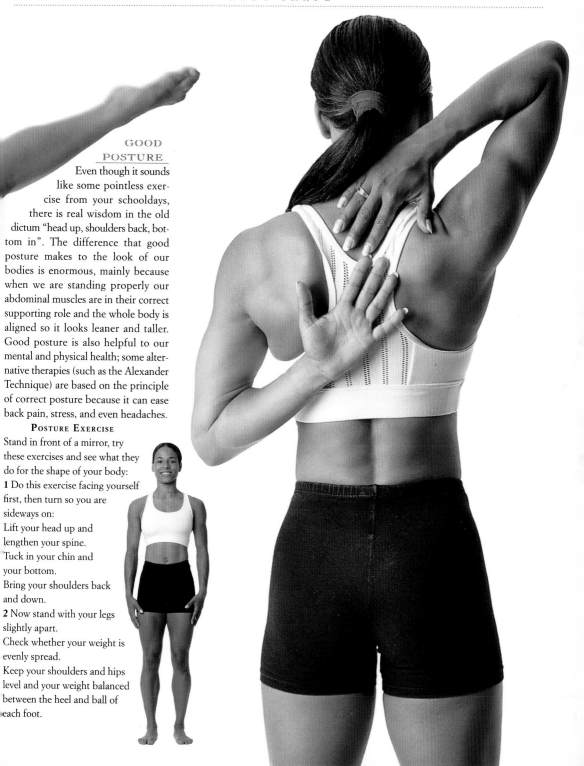

GOOD POSTURE

Even though it sounds like some pointless exercise from your schooldays, there is real wisdom in the old dictum "head up, shoulders back, bottom in". The difference that good posture makes to the look of our bodies is enormous, mainly because when we are standing properly our abdominal muscles are in their correct supporting role and the whole body is aligned so it looks leaner and taller. Good posture is also helpful to our mental and physical health; some alternative therapies (such as the Alexander Technique) are based on the principle of correct posture because it can ease back pain, stress, and even headaches.

POSTURE EXERCISE

Stand in front of a mirror, try these exercises and see what they do for the shape of your body:

1 Do this exercise facing yourself first, then turn so you are sideways on:

Lift your head up and lengthen your spine.

Tuck in your chin and your bottom.

Bring your shoulders back and down.

2 Now stand with your legs slightly apart.

Check whether your weight is evenly spread.

Keep your shoulders and hips level and your weight balanced between the heel and ball of each foot.

TROUBLE SPOTS

Very few people are able to say honestly that they are totally happy with their body. Everyone has at least one gripe – if it is not big feet, it is thin hair or knobbly knees. All these perceived "flaws" can be improved or disguised, but as anyone who has ever tried (and failed) to move the fat that sits on strategic points such as hips, thighs, stomachs, and buttocks knows, it is much easier to hide the flaws than to tackle them. But it is possible to alter your outline with a combination of diet and exercise.

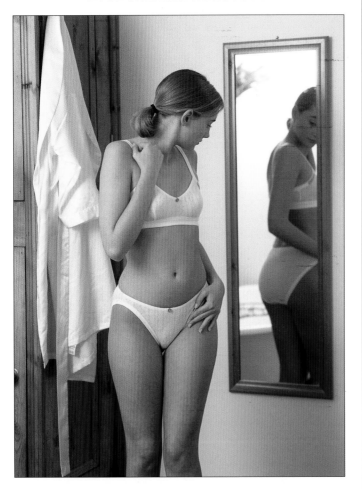

The best way to assess your figure is to stand in front of a full-length mirror. Be honest with yourself, and look for areas that need improving.

FINDING AND IMPROVING YOUR TRUE FORM

Step 1: Confront Your Body
Go on, be brave. Strip to your underwear, stand in front of a mirror and have a good look at your body. Take your time and be tough but realistic. You may have disliked your thighs since you were 16 – and they will probably never be those of a super-model – but if you look hard enough you might just find that they are not as bad as you have always thought they were, and that improving them is not going to be that hard after all.

Step 2: Put Your Complaints in Writing
Note down all the things that irk you (and that you can do something about) as well as those that you like or do not mind. Then go through your list of dislikes, ticking the things that you really want to do something about. Also, make a mental note to start appreciating your good points: the more you focus on them the less you will notice the not-so-good zones.

Step 3: Action Checklist
Now, add a set of action points under the problem zones you have listed. If you want to firm up your arms for that sleeveless sundress you have been unable to wear for a decade of summers, make notes like this:
Flabby Upper Arms
❧ *Do Basic Exercises*
❧ *Check Diet*
❧ *Exfoliate/Moisturize*
Finally, add your goal(s) and your deadline to the top of the list and put it somewhere where you are going to see it frequently.

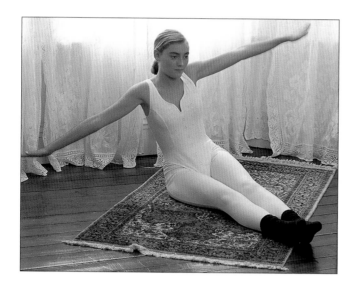

TWO QUICK THIGH-TONERS

If you do not have time to do a full exercise routine, grab 10 minutes in the morning.

Outer Thighs: sit on the floor with your legs straight out in front and hold your arms out to the sides as shown left. Roll sideways on to your bottom – go right over on to your outer thigh and then roll right over on to the other thigh. Do this twenty times.

Inner Thighs: stand upright and consciously tighten – and hold – your buttock muscles for a slow count of 5. Repeat with your thigh muscles and then your calf muscles.

COMMON PROBLEMS

Any of the following can be discouraging, but remember – each problem has a solution.

SLACK STOMACHS

Our stomachs become flabby when the abdominal muscles slacken; this usually happens through lack of exercise. Your abdomen extends from just under the bustline to the groin, and it is packed with muscles that criss-cross to form a wall to hold the abdominal contents in place – a bit like a corset. Exercise is not the only way to keep your stomach flat: weight is also important and the long-term answer is diet and exercise.

THUNDER THIGHS

Thigh size and tone can certainly be altered with the right diet, correct body care and regular exercise. Sports such as cycling, skiing, tennis, squash, and riding (a great inner-muscle firmer) will tone your thighs, as will weight training for specific areas of the body.

LARGE BOTTOMS

There are three large muscles in our buttocks: *gluteus maximus, medius,* and *minimus*. These create the shape, but not the size, of our rear ends. It is the tone of these muscles and the fatty tis-

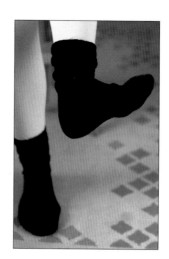

sue around them that gives us the bottoms we have. The good news is that buttock muscles respond well to exercise, which means that any effort you put into bottom-toning exercises will be rewarded quite quickly.

ANKLE EXERCISES

Whenever you remember move your ankles around in a clockwise motion ten times, then repeat anticlockwise.

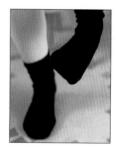

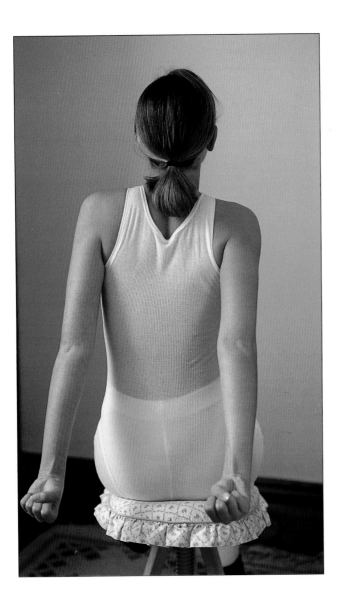

FLABBY ARM FIXER

To firm up flabby arms, add this exercise to your daily exercise routine, or spend five minutes doing it twice a day. Sit on a chair holding your hands in loose fists, and, with your arms extended out behind, make downwards punching movements backwards and forwards.

SLACK UPPER ARMS

Our arms do not really change shape much during our lives, unless we lose or gain a lot of weight. Muscle tone is the main problem, but, as in the case of thighs, exercise and specific weight training will tone up and re-shape flabby arms; very often, any changes in body shape that happen through exercise and diet are noticeable most quickly on your upper arms.

DROOPY BREASTS

Breast shape and size only really change when our weight swings dramatically, or during pregnancy, breast-feeding, menstruation, or if taking oral contraceptives. Gravity is the bust's enemy, especially if the breasts are not given proper support, because it literally drags the breasts down and slackens their tone. Although the breasts are supported by suspension ligaments, they do not contain any muscle (the milk glands are buffered by protective fatty tissue) so you cannot noticeably reverse lost tone. However, if you exercise the pectoral muscles beneath your armpits, you will give your breasts a firmer base and more uplift.

THICK ANKLES

Trim and slender ankles that seem set to snap with every step are a great asset. But if you are not blessed with these, or if your ankles tend to become stiff and puffy from fluid retention, you need to master the art of deception and brush up on some ankle improving exercises.

Assess the flexibility of your ankles by sitting on a chair or stool with your feet on the floor and, while keeping your heel down, pull the rest of your foot up as far as it will go: if the distance between your foot and floor measures 12–15 cm (5–6 in) your joint flexibility is good; if it is between 10–12 cm (4–5 in) it is fair; and if it is less than that, your joint flexibility is poor.

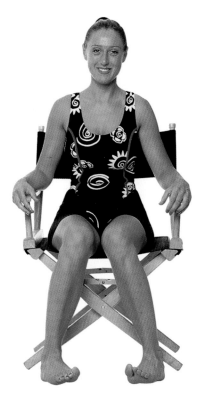

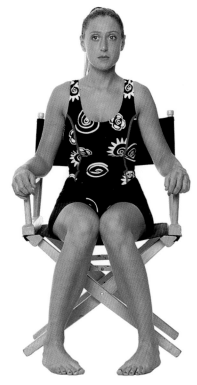

ANKLES AND CALF MUSCLES

EXERCISE A

1 Sit up straight on a chair, with your knees together and heels on the floor and slightly apart, in line with your hips. Bring your big toes up and roll your feet in towards each other.

2 Now tilt and move both feet down and outwards from the ankle, keeping your big toes raised as much as possible as you roll your feet on to their outer edges. Repeat ten times.

EXERCISE B

1 Lie flat on your back on the floor with your legs straight.

2 Bring one leg up and hold it beneath the back of your thigh so that it is pulled towards your chest. Rotate your foot ten times in a clockwise direction and ten times anti-clockwise. Repeat with the other leg. Increase the number of repeats to twenty for each foot, working alternatively in groups of 7.

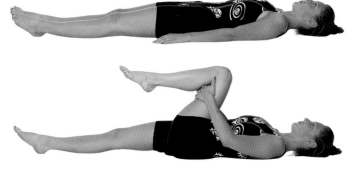

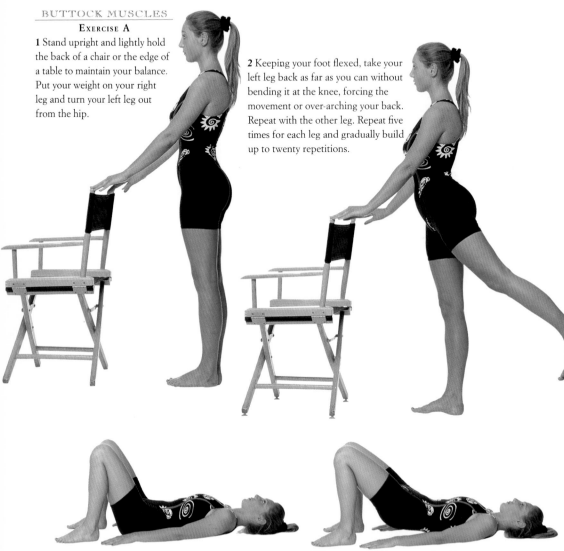

BUTTOCK MUSCLES

EXERCISE A

1 Stand upright and lightly hold the back of a chair or the edge of a table to maintain your balance. Put your weight on your right leg and turn your left leg out from the hip.

2 Keeping your foot flexed, take your left leg back as far as you can without bending it at the knee, forcing the movement or over-arching your back. Repeat with the other leg. Repeat five times for each leg and gradually build up to twenty repetitions.

EXERCISE B

1 Lie on your back with your knees bent and your feet slightly apart, in line with your hips. Place your arms by your sides, palms flat on the floor.

2 Place your weight on your shoulders and upper back (not your neck), raise your bottom and tighten your buttock muscles, keeping your feet flat on the floor and your arms by your sides. Hold for several seconds. Lower your bottom to the floor. Repeat five times, building up to twenty repetitions.

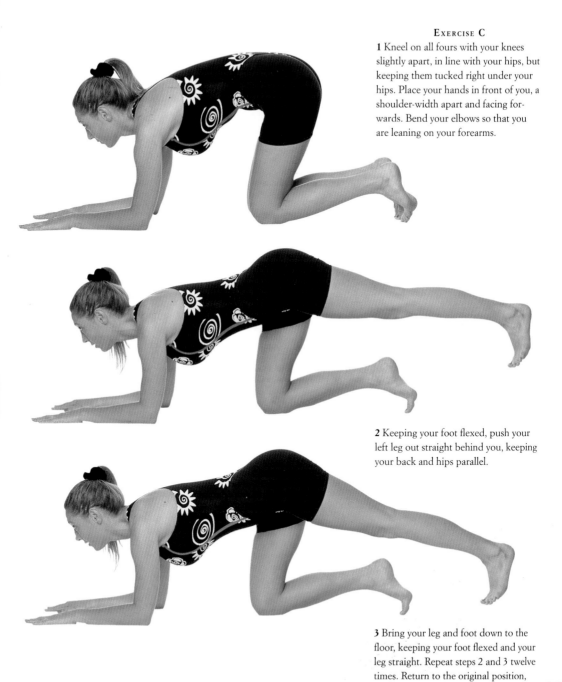

EXERCISE C

1 Kneel on all fours with your knees slightly apart, in line with your hips, but keeping them tucked right under your hips. Place your hands in front of you, a shoulder-width apart and facing forwards. Bend your elbows so that you are leaning on your forearms.

2 Keeping your foot flexed, push your left leg out straight behind you, keeping your back and hips parallel.

3 Bring your leg and foot down to the floor, keeping your foot flexed and your leg straight. Repeat steps 2 and 3 twelve times. Return to the original position, then repeat the exercise with your other leg. Build up to twenty repetitions.

GLOSSARY

ACUTE CONDITION: Arising suddenly and with intense severity, but only running a short course. (See chronic condition)

ALLOPATHIC: The conventional method of combating disease by using active ingredients specifically against the disease.

ANAEMIA: A deficiency in red blood cells, or in the haemoglobin carried by them. The resultant lack of oxygen carried around the body produces pallor, breathlessness and no energy.

ANALGESIC: Relieves pain.

APERIENT: A mild laxative.

ATROPHY: The shrinking or wasting away of muscles, glands or tissues due to disease or malnutrition.

BILE: A bitter green to brown alkaline fluid produced by the liver and stored in the gall bladder.

BILIOUS: Any disorder which results in the production of an excess amount of bile.

CHRONIC CONDITION: A disease or ailment that develops slowly and persists over a long period of time. (See acute condition)

DEMULCENT: Oily substance used to soften and soothe damaged surfaces such as the skin, or mucous membranes.

DILUENT: A substance used for dilution, e.g. water, base oil.

DIURETIC: Encourages urination.

DYSPEPSIA: Indigestion.

EMETIC: Causes vomiting.

EMOLLIENT: Softens and soothes the skin.

ENDOGENOUS: Caused or produced by factors within the organism or system.

FEBRIFUGE: Reduces fever.

FEBRILE: Feverish, or relating to a fever.

FIBROIDS: A structure resembling or consisting of fibrous tissue.

FOMENTATION: The act of applying heat and moisture to relieve inflammation and pain.

LEUCORRHEA: White to yellowish vaginal discharge.

MUCOUS MEMBRANE: Soft tissue lining most of the body's cavities and tubes.

PAROXYSMAL: A sudden attack or occurrence of a disease.

PERISTALSIS: Waves of contractions passing along the walls of hollow muscular organs, forcing the contents forwards.

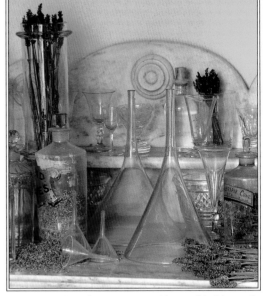

PHARMACOPOEIA: An authoritative written guide to medicinal drugs and their uses.

PROGESTERONE: A natural hormone that prepares the uterus to receive and develop the fertilized egg.

PROPHYLACTIC: Preventing or protecting from disease.

SALICYLATES: Salts of salicylic acid.

SALICYLIC ACID: A white crystalline substance used in the manufacture of aspirin.

SUCCUSS: A special way of shaking a homeopathic remedy in order to extract its medicinal properties.

SUPPURATING: Oozing.

SYNOVIAL MEMBRANE: Soft tissues lining joints and tendon sheaths.

TONIC: Invigorates and tones the body and promotes well-being.

TRIGEMINAL NERVES: Either of the fifth pair of cranial nerves which supply the muscles of the upper and lower jawbone.

WATERBRASH: Gas being brought up into the mouth with acidic fluid.

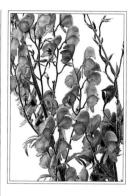

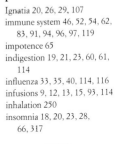
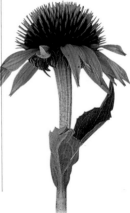

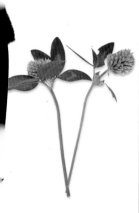

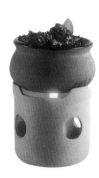

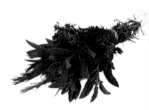

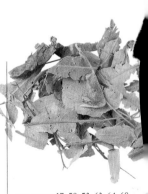

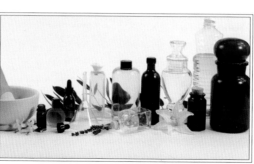

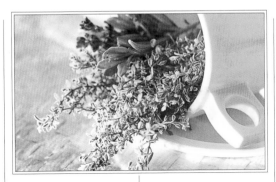